CAMBRIDGE LIBRARY COLLECTION

Books of enduring scholarly value

History of Medicine

It is sobering to realise that as recently as the year in which On the Origin of Species was published, learned opinion was that diseases such as typhus and cholera were spread by a 'miasma', and suggestions that doctors should wash their hands before examining patients were greeted with mockery by the profession. The Cambridge Library Collection reissues milestone publications in the history of Western medicine as well as studies of other medical traditions. Its coverage ranges from Galen on anatomical procedures to Florence Nightingale's common-sense advice to nurses, and includes early research into genetics and mental health, colonial reports on tropical diseases, documents on public health and military medicine, and publications on spa culture and medicinal plants.

A Treatise on Pulmonary Consumption

Having trained in Edinburgh as a surgeon and served aboard Royal Navy vessels, Sir James Clark (1788–1870) developed a particular interest in the spread of the tuberculosis pandemic in Europe. A licentiate of the Royal College of Physicians from 1826, and elected to the Royal Society in 1832, he became a trusted physician and friend to Queen Victoria and Prince Albert. This influential work of 1835 focuses on the treatment and prevention of tuberculosis. Written for a general as well as medical readership, it was lauded by *The Lancet* and ran to several English editions along with translations into other languages. Also reissued in this series are Clark's *Medical Notes on Climate, Diseases, Hospitals, and Medical Schools in France, Italy, and Switzerland* (1820), *The Influence of Climate in the Prevention and Cure of Chronic Diseases* (1829) and his *Memoir of John Conolly* (1869).

Cambridge University Press has long been a pioneer in the reissuing of out-of-print titles from its own backlist, producing digital reprints of books that are still sought after by scholars and students but could not be reprinted economically using traditional technology. The Cambridge Library Collection extends this activity to a wider range of books which are still of importance to researchers and professionals, either for the source material they contain, or as landmarks in the history of their academic discipline.

Drawing from the world-renowned collections in the Cambridge University Library and other partner libraries, and guided by the advice of experts in each subject area, Cambridge University Press is using state-of-the-art scanning machines in its own Printing House to capture the content of each book selected for inclusion. The files are processed to give a consistently clear, crisp image, and the books finished to the high quality standard for which the Press is recognised around the world. The latest print-on-demand technology ensures that the books will remain available indefinitely, and that orders for single or multiple copies can quickly be supplied.

The Cambridge Library Collection brings back to life books of enduring scholarly value (including out-of-copyright works originally issued by other publishers) across a wide range of disciplines in the humanities and social sciences and in science and technology.

A Treatise on
Pulmonary Consumption

Comprehending an Inquiry into the Causes,
Nature, Prevention and Treatment of Tuberculous
and Scrofulous Diseases in General

JAMES CLARK

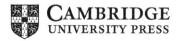

CAMBRIDGE
UNIVERSITY PRESS

CAMBRIDGE
UNIVERSITY PRESS

University Printing House, Cambridge, CB2 8BS, United Kingdom

Published in the United States of America by Cambridge University Press, New York

Cambridge University Press is part of the University of Cambridge.

It furthers the University's mission by disseminating knowledge in the pursuit of education, learning and research at the highest international levels of excellence.

www.cambridge.org
Information on this title: www.cambridge.org/9781108062305

© in this compilation Cambridge University Press 2013

This edition first published 1835
This digitally printed version 2013

ISBN 978-1-108-06230-5 Paperback

A

TREATISE

ON

PULMONARY CONSUMPTION

COMPREHENDING

AN INQUIRY INTO

THE

CAUSES NATURE PREVENTION

AND

TREATMENT

OF

TUBERCULOUS AND SCROFULOUS DISEASES

IN GENERAL

———————

By JAMES CLARK, M.D. F.R.S.

CONSULTING PHYSICIAN TO THEIR MAJESTIES THE KING AND QUEEN OF THE
BELGIANS AND PHYSICIAN IN ORDINARY TO THEIR ROYAL HIGHNESSES
THE DUCHESS OF KENT AND THE PRINCESS VICTORIA.

———————

LONDON

SHERWOOD GILBERT AND PIPER

PATERNOSTER-ROW.

———

M DCCC XXXV

Treatise for your Majesty's gracious acceptance; and when I reflect that the object of my humble labours is to inculcate doctrines of infinite importance to the health of mankind and the general well-being of society, I feel an anxious desire that it may be found not undeserving of a patronage so high and so influential.

It is only by convincing the public of the comparative futility of all attempts to cure consumption, and of the signal efficacy of proper measures directed to prevent it, that physicians can ever hope to produce those beneficial results in improving public health and in preserving and prolonging human life, which it is the distinguishing privilege of their profession to aim at. And in looking to your Majesty in your elevated station and high character—the chosen and beloved sovereign of a great and free people—I cannot contemplate a higher fortune for my book, or one more likely to secure the object with which it was composed, than that of its obtaining the approbation and protection of your Majesty.

That your Majesty may long enjoy the happiness to reign in the hearts of a prosperous and loyal people is the fervent prayer of

Your Majesty's

Most grateful and devoted servant,

JAMES CLARK.

LONDON, JUNE 1835.

PREFACE.

THE greater part of the following Treatise first appeared as an article in the Cyclopædia of Practical Medicine, under the head of TUBERCULAR PHTHISIS. In publishing it as a separate work various alterations and additions were required : these I have endeavoured to supply as fully as the short space of time which has elapsed since its first appearance permitted. That the work might have been rendered more perfect by deferring its publication I readily admit; but after mature consideration I venture to lay it before the public without further delay.

If I am not greatly deceived, the view which I have taken of tuberculous diseases is calculated to lead to a more successful method, both of prevention and treatment, than has hitherto prevailed. With this impression on my mind I feel myself justified in submitting my views and opinions to the consideration of the profession,—well aware, that, if erroneous, the task of correcting them is not very likely to originate with their author, and that, if well founded, the efforts of an individual can avail little in procuring the general application of them.

Although I have entered more particularly into the history of tuberculous disease of the lungs, or pulmonary consumption, my observations will be found to be applicable to the whole class of tuberculous and scrofulous diseases. They all originate in the same constitutional disorder, acknowledge the same remote causes, and admit of the same rules of prevention ; and, I may add, that the same mode of treatment is essentially applicable to the whole.

The total inefficacy of all means hitherto adopted for diminishing the frequency or reducing the mortality of this class of diseases, is of itself sufficient incitement to us to seek for some other method of remedying the evil ; and it is evident to me that this can only be done, with any reasonable prospect of success, by directing the attention to such measures as are calculated to prevent the hereditary transmission of the particular morbid state in which the formal disease originates, and to correct the predisposition to it in infancy and youth. It is, accordingly, on this part of my subject, which involves the consideration of the Origin, Causes, and Prevention of the disease, that I have more especially dwelt.

I cannot but be aware of the great difficulties which present themselves to the accomplishment of my views regarding Prevention ; and that these can, never become generally applicable until the public is fully impressed with the necessity of attending to them. This furnishes me with another urgent

motive for the publication of the present
work ; as it is only by the combined exertions of the profession that the public can
be influenced in such a case. And here I
hope I may be allowed to calculate the more
surely on the support of my medical brethren,
because, in setting forth my views and opinions,
I make no pretension to originality or peculiarity of doctrine. Much that is contained
in the following pages is already known to
the more intelligent and experienced of the
profession, and the only credit I can claim, is
the having, perhaps, placed the subject in a
more striking point of view, and advocated it
with a degree of earnestness commensurate
with its importance.

The subject, in the comprehensive view
which I have taken of it, involves so many
momentous considerations, and embraces so
wide a range, that some points deserving
notice may, no doubt, have escaped me,
while others may be regarded as too lightly
treated : still I trust it will be found that

I have omitted nothing of real importance. If zeal for the accomplishment of my main object has induced me to enter into and dwell more fully upon some parts than others, the conviction of their paramount importance must be my apology. My great aim has been to point out the nature and causes of the constitutional affection in which tuberculous diseases have their origin, and on those to found rules for prevention and treatment.

By diminishing the disposition to this most destructive of all human maladies, we shall not only reduce the sum of its daily victims, but we shall raise the standard of public health, and at the same time advance the moral excellence of man, augment his mental capabilities, and increase the sphere of his usefulness ; for it need not be stated, that without sound bodily health, the intellectual powers languish and decay. Our subject, therefore, is one which not only concerns personal feelings and social happiness, but involves the well-being of society at large, and the intellectual as well as the physical character of nations. And when we further consider that the disposition to tuberculous diseases, and the deterioration of health which this implies, are evidently, to me at least, on the increase, assuredly no higher object than that to which the present work is devoted can engage the attention of the physician; and if I succeed in awakening a more general interest in the profession towards it, and in pointing out a surer path for observation, I shall not have laboured in vain.

Respecting the alterations which have been made in my work since its original publication, I may state that the whole has been carefully revised, much the greater part re-written, and considerable additions made to almost every chapter; more particularly to those on the Causes and Prevention. But I am fully sensible that much is still wanting to illustrate this the most important part of

the subject, and that the labours of many
men and of many years will be required to
complete a work which I consider as only
just begun.

I may further state that I have avoided
entering into theoretical discussions ; my object being to adhere, as closely as the nature
of the subject would admit, to the simple
results of observation, and what appeared to
be legitimate deductions from them. There
being also a probability that my work, from
the importance and general interest of the
subject, may pass into the hands of the public,
I have endeavoured to divest my language
as much as possible of technical terms.

LONDON, JUNE 30, 1835.

BY THE SAME AUTHOR, SECOND EDITION,

A TREATISE

ON THE

INFLUENCE OF CLIMATE

IN THE

PREVENTION AND CURE

OF

CHRONIC DISEASES OF THE CHEST,
DIGESTIVE ORGANS, ETC.

CONTENTS.

b

CHAP. III.

PARTICULAR SYMPTOMS AND SIGNS OF CONSUMPTION. 69

CHAP. IV.

MORBID ANATOMY OF TUBERCULOUS DISEASE. 118

CHAP. V.

CURE OF TUBERCULOUS DISEASE OF THE LUNGS 137

CHAP. VI.

DISEASES WHICH ATTEND AND COMPLICATE
CONSUMPTION   144

CHAP. VII.

DURATION OF CONSUMPTION   .   . 165

CHAP. VIII.

STATISTICAL HISTORY OF CONSUMPTION 170

CHAP. IX.

TUBERCULOUS DISEASES IN ANIMALS 212

CHAP. X.

CAUSES OF TUBERCULOUS DISEASE . 219

CHAP. XI.

PATHOLOGY OF CONSUMPTION AND OF
TUBERCULOUS DISEASES IN GENERAL .

CHAP. XII.

PREVENTION OF CONSUMPTION AND OF
TUBERCULOUS DISEASES IN GENERAL .

A

TREATISE

ON

PULMONARY CONSUMPTION,

ETC. ETC.

INTRODUCTION.

THE term Phthisis, or Consumption, was originally applied in a very vague manner to a variety
of chronic diseases, having scarcely any character
in common except emaciation. As the knowledge
of morbid anatomy became more precise, the most
frequent cause of the phenomena usually grouped
under the name of Consumption, was discovered to
be disease of the lungs, and hence pulmonary
consumption not only attracted far greater attention
than any other form of the disease, but many
of the other forms were found to resolve themselves into this, or to be mere complications of it;
the primary cause of the emaciation and other

B

symptoms, being discovered, on examination after death, to be seated in the lungs. Pulmonary consumption was therefore adopted as the generic name of the disease, and was divided into various species according to the particular affection of the respiratory organs upon which the symptoms were supposed to depend.

At length, Laennec, finding, in the course of his extensive researches into diseases of the chest, that tubercles formed almost the sole cause of consumption, proposed to restrict the term Phthisis to the disease produced by tubercles in the lungs; and since the publication of his valuable work in 1819, which forms an important era in our knowledge of pulmonary pathology, the term has been so restricted in France. The accuracy of Laennec's opinions has been fully confirmed by his countrymen Louis and Andral, whose minute and laborious investigations have given a precision to our knowledge of the subject, which was unattained before their time. But, notwithstanding the great advantages which have resulted from these pathological researches, they have tended to keep up the idea that consumption is a local disease, referable to a local cause; and thus the investigation of the constitutional origin of tubercles,—by far the most important part of the subject,—has been neglected.

Before we can hope to acquire an accurate knowledge of consumption, we must carry our researches beyond the pulmonary disease, which is only a secondary affection, the consequence of a pre-existing constitutional disorder,—the necessary condition which determines the production of tubercles.

An imperfect acquaintance with this morbid state of the system has led to great discrepancy of opinion concerning the nature and causes of tubercles. There are many, even at the present day, who regard tuberculous disease of the lungs as the result of inflammation; an opinion which I regard as not only erroneous, but productive of a very mischievous practice. Inflammation of the respiratory organs may, no doubt, give rise to tubercles, but not, I believe, in a healthy constitution.

Chronic inflammation of the different tissues of which the lungs are composed, is often accompanied with symptoms closely resembling those produced by tuberculous disease; and the distinction between them becomes, in some cases, very difficult,—more especially after the tuberculous disease has existed for some time and become complicated with inflammation. Hence inflammatory and tuberculous diseases have been, and still are often confounded, and even considered by many in the light of cause and effect. This error originates not so much in the nature of the subject, as in a want of correct observation; and I am of opinion

that when such inflammatory affections are carefully traced to their origin, they may, in a very
large proportion of cases, be discriminated from
pure tuberculous disease. That the distinction is
not more frequently made, is owing more to our
own imperfect and careless inquiries into the history of the cases which come before us, and to
our negligence in examining minutely all the signs
and symptoms which they present, than to any
real obscurity in the nature and characters of the
diseases themselves:—The truth is, that in the
highly-tuberculous constitution, tuberculous disease
of the lungs very often steals on in a slow, insidious
manner, making considerable progress before it
manifests itself by any remarkable local symptoms,
or its existence is even suspected by those who
regard consumption as originating in inflammatory
affections of the lungs. In such examples of latent
tuberculous disease, an attack of catarrh, a slight
inflammation of the pleura, or of the lungs, or
hemoptysis, is not unfrequently the first circumstance
which excites the attention or awakens the fears of
the patient and his friends; and to this accidental
occurrence, to which the presence of tubercles in
the lungs renders the person peculiarly liable, the
origin of all the future mischief is attributed.
I can readily imagine that an ordinary observer
should arrive at such a conclusion; and, ascribing
the disease to that which first presented itself to

his notice, should consider the 'neglected cold,' the 'inflammation of the lungs,' or the 'breaking of a bloodvessel,' the original cause and source of all the subsequent evil. But, after the light which has of late been thrown upon the nature and diagnosis of tuberculous disease, it may well excite surprise that medical men should still regard these affections as the chief causes of Phthisis. In a vast proportion of cases of this nature, a more minute inquiry into the patient's previous state of health, would have led to the conviction that those affections were consequent upon, or at least subsequent to, the existence of pulmonary tubercles, or that they had occurred in a tuberculous constitution, by which their effects were modified. In another part of this treatise I shall have occasion to state the grounds upon which this opinion rests, and at the same time shall endeavour to show that tuberculous disease of the lungs may be detected long before it generally is,—that what is usually considered the early is in reality an advanced stage of the disease,—and that tubercle is a secondary affection, originating in a peculiar morbid condition of the general system.

One of the principal objects of the present work is to shew that tuberculous disease, whether in the lungs or elsewhere, has its origin in a morbid state of the constitution, in some cases hereditary, in others induced from various causes, independent of any hereditary predisposition; and to attach the proper value to those pulmonary diseases which are considered by some as the real causes of consumption, but by others, more correctly, as determining causes merely, and often only complications.

If I succeed in giving a satisfactory exposition of this, the most important, but hitherto the most neglected part of the subject, I may hope to lay the foundation of a sounder pathology of tuberculous diseases, and to establish a more rational and more effectual mode of prevention, and a more successful method of treatment than has hitherto prevailed. No physician, acquainted with the morbid anatomy of Tuberculous Consumption, can for a moment indulge the hope that we shall ever be able to cure what is usually termed ' confirmed consumption,' if we except the small proportion of cases in which the tuberculous deposit is confined to a very limited portion of the lung. We might as reasonably expect to restore vision when the organization of the eye is destroyed, or the functions of the brain when the substance of that organ is reduced by disease to a pultaceous mass, as to cure a patient whose lungs are extensively disorganized by tuberculous disease. The records of Medicine afford too strong proofs of the truth of this statement; for it may be fairly questioned whether the proportion of cures of confirmed consumption is greater at the present day than in the time of Hippocrates; and, although the public may continue to be the dupes of boasting charlatans, I am persuaded that no essential progress has been made, or can be made in the cure of consumption, until the disease is treated upon different principles from what it hitherto has been. If the labour and ingenuity which have been misapplied in fruitless attempts to cure an irremediable condition of the lungs, had been rightly directed to the investigation of the causes and nature of tuberculous disease, the subject of our inquiry would have been regarded in a very different light from that in which it is at the present period.

By a knowledge of the causes of the morbid condition of the system in which tuberculous disease has its origin, we may reasonably hope to prevent the occurrence of the latter in many cases, and in a small proportion to arrest its progress during the early stage; and by carrying our researches still further back and investigating the circumstances in the health of the parents which predispose their offspring to tuberculous disease, we may also hope to diminish the hereditary disposition. This is, no doubt, opening a very wide field of inquiry; but it is most certain that, unless we enter into the subject in its fullest extent, we shall do little that will prove effectual in diminishing the frequency, or reducing the mortality of this very prevalent and most destructive malady.

In the long catalogue of human infirmities, tuber-

culous diseases are undoubtedly the most deserving
the study of the physician, whether we regard their
frequency or mortality. Confined to no country,
age, sex, or condition of life, they destroy a larger
proportion of mankind in temperate climates than
all other chronic diseases taken together. In this
country, and over the whole temperate region of
Europe and America, tuberculous disease of the
lungs causes probably a fifth-part of the whole mortality; and in some districts, and even in whole
countries, the proportion is much larger. It has
been calculated by the late Dr. Young, Dr. Wooll-
combe, and others, from the best data which the
bills of mortality afford, that in Great Britain and
Ireland, consumption causes one fourth-part of the
deaths that occur from disease. If we add to consumption, tuberculous disease of the glandular and
nervous systems, of the large joints, of the spinal
column, &c. and deduct the mortality which occurs
during the first months of life, I shall probably be
within the truth in stating that a third-part of the
mortality of this country arises from tuberculous
diseases: if to this frightful destruction of mankind
we add the numerous crippled and disfigured
sufferers whom we daily meet with, and couple
these results with the painful reflection that
the predisposition to tuberculous diseases is transmitted from the parent to the offspring, it will
surely be unnecessary to press upon medical prac-

titioners the claim which this class of diseases, above all others, has upon their earnest consideration.

The subject considered in this comprehensive manner possesses a degree of importance unquestionably beyond any other in the whole range of medical science : and I do not hesitate to express my conviction that in proportion as the medical practitioner is acquainted with the remote and exciting causes of tuberculous disease, so will he be enabled to treat successfully a large number of the diseases which come under his care : this remark applies more especially to the diseases of of childhood and youth,—for it is during this early period of life that tuberculous disease is so easily generated, and that so much may be done to destroy the hereditary tendency to it.

To those who have not maturely considered this subject in all its bearings, I may appear to attach too much importance to it; but I feel confident, nevertheless, that my opinions will be borne out by future inquirers, and by those of my professional brethren who are best acquainted with human pathology.

A very important question in the history of tuberculous diseases naturally presents itself to our consideration in this place, viz. their increasing or decreasing frequency. Every member of the profession has too ample opportunities of satisfying

himself of the extensive prevalence of strumous
diseases; but some doubts may exist as to their
being comparatively more prevalent at the present
time than they were some fifty or a hundred years
ago. The labouring classes of this country are
certainly in the enjoyment of more comfort in
regard to their food, clothing, and lodging, at the
present period than they were half a century back;
but although this circumstance favours the probability of a diminution of tuberculous diseases, it
may be doubted whether such abatement has not
been counteracted by the more general indulgence
in the use of ardent spirits which prevails at present
among this class of the people.* But whether
tuberculous diseases have diminished or not during
the last half century among the labouring part of
our population, I am of opinion that they have
increased in the middle and upper ranks. This is
a subject of great moment. If it were clearly shown
that these diseases were gradually abating among
all ranks of the people, we might perhaps leave them
in the hope that their diminution would keep pace
with the improvement of society. But if, on the
contrary, we arrive at the conclusion that scrofulous
diseases are on the increase, and that the health of the
middle and upper ranks of society is progressively

---

* This subject will be treated more fully in the chapter on the
STATISTICS OF CONSUMPTION.

declining, we shall have the strongest reasons for inquiring into the causes which lead to such deterioration of health.

That a general delicacy of constitution and a proneness to scrofulous diseases are on the increase, is a conclusion the accuracy of which I leave to be decided by the experience of the profession.* We have all an opportunity of observing and comparing the state of health of the rising generation with that of their fathers and grandfathers. On taking a survey of the constitution of these three generations, I think it will be found, in a large proportion of instances, that the deterioration of health is progressive from father to son. I am far from believing that this observation always holds good; but I do believe that it generally does: at least, such is the conclusion to which I have been led from personal observation.

* The terms *Scrofulous* and *Strumous,* when strictly applied, have the same import as *Tuberculous,* and are used in this sense in the following pages.

CHAPTER I.

TUBERCULOUS CACHEXIA.

As I shall have frequent occasion, in the course of the present work, to refer to that morbid condition of the system which precedes and attends tuberculous disease, I shall commence by giving a brief view of the characters by which it may generally be recognised. It is proper, however, to premise that, although distinct and sufficiently recognisable, these characters are so variously influenced by the age, complexion, temperament, and other circumstances of the individual, as to make it a matter of considerable difficulty to describe them. It must also be observed that the morbid condition upon which they depend is itself progressive, and therefore varies in intensity.

By the term TUBERCULOUS CACHEXIA, I designate that particular morbid condition of the system which gives rise to the deposition of tuberculous matter, on the application of certain exciting causes, which have no such effect on a healthy system. This disorder of the constitution, noticed by various authors under different names, (latent scrofula, scrofulous diathesis, &c.,) was, I believe, first described under the present appellation in my work on CLIMATE.*

Tuberculous Cachexia may exist from birth, or may be acquired at almost any period of life, from infancy to old age. When of hereditary origin, it is manifested by a peculiar modification of the whole organization,—in structure and in form, in action and in function.

The countenance generally affords strong indications of the presence of this affection; in early childhood it has a pale, pasty appearance, the cheeks are generally full, and the upper lip and nose tumid. If the complexion be dark, the colour of the skin is generally sallow; if fair, it has an unnatural white appearance, resembling blanched wax rather than healthy integument; and the veins are large and conspicuous. At a more advanced period of youth, the character of the constitution is still more clearly indicated by the countenance. The eyes, particularly the pupils, are generally large, the eye-lashes long; and there is usually a placid expression, often great beauty of countenance, especially in persons of a fair, florid complexion. On the other hand, in those of a dark complexion, the features are generally less regular,

---

* " The INFLUENCE OF CLIMATE in the Prevention and Cure of Chronic Diseases of the Chest, &c."

and the skin is commonly coarse, and of a sallow, dingy hue; although there are many exceptions to this, in the fine dark eye, regular features, and delicate skin of such persons. But it is far more easy to distinguish than to describe with accuracy the tuberculous physiognomy, as it varies in every intermediate shade, between the pale, faded, but changing colour of persons little under the influence of this morbid condition, and the peculiar permanent sallow cast of countenance which attends the confirmed cachectic state.

In early infancy there is little remarkable in the form of the body; it is generally large, but has not the firmness of health. As the child increases in age, we find that the different parts are not well proportioned, and there is a want of symmetry in the whole. The head is often large, the trunk small, the abdomen tumid, and the limbs are unshapely, being either large and clumsy, or disproportionately slender with large joints: but this is only the case in the more perfect examples of hereditary tuberculous cachexia. The growth of the body is also generally unsteady in its progress; very often it is slowly and imperfectly developed; in other cases it is unusually rapid, particularly towards puberty.

Thenphysical powers are generally below the usual standard. The limbs, though full, are soft, and have neither the form nor the firmness of health.

The circulation is generally feeble, as is indicated by a weak pulse and cold extremities. This state of the circulating system forms, I am disposed to believe, an element in the tuberculous constitution; at least I have rarely found it wanting, and regard it as affording an explanation of many of the phenomena of the disease. A full development of the body and great muscular power are not, however, incompatible with a degree of tuberculous cachexia. Several of our celebrated pugilists have died tuberculous. Independently of their bearing on the present subject, such examples deserve attention, as showing the effect of training in increasing the strength even of the tuberculous system.

The functions of organic life are all more or less imperfectly performed, but those more immediately connected with nutrition, particularly the digestive function, are most evidently deranged. Digestion is rarely well performed; the bowels are irregular, more frequently slow in their action than the reverse, and the evacuations have not the appearance which they are known to possess in health. The urinary secretion, also, deviates from the healthy characters, being commonly turbid, particularly when the bowels are costive. The cutaneous functions are very generally in an unhealthy state; the skin is either soft and flaccid, or dry and harsh, and chronic eruptions of the dry, scaly cha-

racter, are frequent. In general the insensible perspiration is defective, although copious partial perspirations are common, particularly on the feet,
where they often have a fetid odour. But of all
these disordered functions, that which claims our
principal attention, because it is the primary one,
and from it arise most of the others, is the disorder of the digestive organs. The dyspepsia of
the tuberculous constitution has peculiar characters
by which it may generally be known. These have
been fully and accurately described by Dr. Todd,
under the name of *Strumous Dyspepsia;** a condition of the digestive organs which is not only
present in the hereditary strumous constitution,
but is capable, I believe, of generating this constitution, and of leading ultimately to tuberculous
cachexia. In Dr. Todd's opinion, " it presents a
more characteristic feature of this habit of body
than any physiognomical portrait which has yet
been drawn of it. In this respect it is more to be
depended on than either the fine skin, the clear,
delicate complexion, the light hair, large blue
eyes, and dull sclerotica of one variety; or the
foul, dull, swarthy-coloured skin, the sallow complexion and swollen countenance, the dark hair and
tumid lip of the other. It betokens, indeed, little
familiarity with scrofula to connect it with any

* See his admirable article on INDIGESTION, in the second
volume of *The Cyclopædia of Practical Medicine.*

particular temperament, for it belongs to all temperaments,—to the sanguine as well as the phleg-
matic, to the nervous as well as the melancholic,
and to all their varieties and combinations. But
upon whatever temperament the disordered habit
which we call scrofula may engraft itself, we venture to say that this form of dyspepsia will also
there be found; and, therefore, being constantly
present with it, preceding and accompanying the
various symptoms which issue from it, it would be
contrary to all reason to refuse to it an important
share in the development of this disordered habit,
and in the production of the local affections which
have hitherto too much engrossed the attention, to
the exclusion of a proper consideration of the constitutional disease." I have great pleasure and
satisfaction in citing Dr. Todd's observations, because they are in accordance with my own, and
because they cannot, in my opinion, be too strongly
pressed upon the consideration of the profession;
so much importance do I attach to this disordered
state of the digestive organs as a source of tuberculous disease.

I shall now notice the leading symptoms by which
this affection of the digestive organs is characc-
terized,—more especially in children, in whom
it is so important to attend to it. The tongue is
redder than natural, especially towards the extremity and along the margins; the anterior part is

thickly spotted with small red points of a still brighter colour, the central portion being more or less furred, in general according to the duration of the disorder; sometimes the tongue is covered with a dirty whitish fur, through which the red papillæ project; in which case the central part of the tongue is often dry and of a brownish colour in the morning. There is generally some thirst: the appetite is variable, more frequently craving than deficient, seldom natural; and the breath is fetid. The bowels are generally confined, though occasionally they are too loose; the evacuations are always unnatural, generally of a pale, greyish colour, of the consistence and appearance of moist clay; and they are often mixed with mucus and partially digested food. The urine is often turbid, sometimes high-coloured, and at other times too abundant and pale. The skin is generally harsh and dry, or subject to cold perspirations, particularly the hands and feet, which are habitually cold; copious partial night-sweats are common. The sleep is seldom sound,—the child is restless, and talks in his sleep, or grinds his teeth.

When this disordered state has continued for some time, the complexion loses its natural colour, and the face has a pasty, faded aspect; the child is languid, disinclined for exercise or play, and generally fretful; a train of secondary disorders also soon appears, as a consequence of the irritation

of the digestive organs. The internal fauces become full and red, inflammatory sore-throats are
common, and the tonsils often become permanently
enlarged. The nose is generally dry, or discharges
thick mucus in large quantity; and epistaxis occasionally occurs. The eye-lids are subject to chronic inflammation; and eruptions behind the ears
and on the scalp, or other parts, are very frequent.
Copious discharges of mucus, sometimes mixed
with blood, take place from the bowels, and from
the bronchial membrane; and are indeed common
from all the mucous surfaces. The brain and spinal
marrow frequently become the seat of secondary
irritation, and hydrocephalus, epilepsy, and chorea,
or paralysis may be the consequence; but the most
frequent and most important of all the consequences
of this disordered state of the digestive organs is
tuberculous cachexia.

The above may be considered a summary of the
symptoms and progress of Strumous or Tuberculous Dyspepsia. This disorder has been no where,
or at least so well, described, as in the Essay
by Dr. Todd already referred to. It is scarcely
known, and yet without a knowledge of it no
one can understand the treatment of scrofulous
disease, in any of its forms. On this account
I would strongly recommend the study of the characters of Strumous Dyspepsia to the younger
members of the profession.

The state of the nervous system in Tuberculous
Cachexia varies greatly in different individuals; it
is generally morbidly sensitive and irritable: in persons naturally of a nervous temperament, more especially females, the nervous sensibility is greatly
increased. The intellectual functions are often performed with a preternatural degree of activity, a
premature development of the mental faculties
being a frequent accompaniment of the tuberculous
habit;—a circumstance which demands our attention,
on account of the practical rules to be founded on it,
in regulating the education of such persons. But
this state of the intellect is by no means a constant
attendant on the scrofulous constitution; indeed,
the very reverse often prevails. We meet with two
opposite states of the mental as well as physical constitution: the one, attended by a florid complexion,
thin, fair skin, and great sensibility to impressions,
with a corresponding acuteness of mind ; the other,
characterized by a dark complexion and coarse skin,
with a languid, torpid condition of the bodily
functions, and a similar dulness of the mental faculties.

When Tuberculous Cachexia is acquired later in
life, the characters by which it is recognized are
less clearly marked and less easily distinguished,
than when it occurs as an hereditary affection, or
is engrafted on the tuberculous constitution. We
want in a great degree the external features and

form which characterize the hereditary disease. But even when cachexia has been acquired after maturity, the peculiar pallid hue, approaching to sallow, and the sunk and faded state of the features, are in general sufficiently well-marked to indicate the patient's condition. In persons of dark complexion there is an unvarying sallow, or rather leaden hue of the skin, and a dull pearly appearance of the sclerotica; and in the fair and florid, a pasty aspect of the countenance, alternating with the irregular red and white mottled appearance of the cheeks, passing often from the paleness of death to a dark purplish hue, in a way more easily recognized than described. In more advanced life, the pale, sallow cast of countenance, varying occasionally to a tinge of yellow, predominates, and marks the slowly acquired but deeply rooted constitutional disease.

CHAPTER II.

TUBERCULOUS DISEASE OF THE LUNGS, OR PUL-
MONARY CONSUMPTION, PROPERLY SO CALLED.

IN describing the course of tuberculous consumption, I shall endeavour to trace the relation between
the symptoms and the physical signs, which attend
and mark the progressive morbid changes in the
lungs; as it is only by keeping this connexion
constantly in view that we are able to detect tuberculous disease in its commencement, follow it in
its course, or distinguish it even in its more
advanced stages, when latent, or obscured by the
presence of other diseases.

Although a certain group of symptoms accompany pulmonary consumption, the order in which
they present themselves and the degree of their
intensity vary remarkably in different individuals.
In some cases the symptoms are so prominent as to
excite the attention of the most careless observer;
while in others they are so slight as scarcely to be
observed by any but the medical attendant, and
they even occasionally escape his observation, until
the disease is far advanced.

I shall, in the first place, describe the more usual form and progress of consumption, and afterwards notice the less common, but not less certain, forms, which it occasionally assumes. I shall also adopt the usual mode of dividing the disease into stages, as it will enable me more easily to follow the progress of the pulmonary affection in connection with its external manifestations.

SECT. I.—THE MORE COMMON OR GENERAL FORM OF CONSUMPTION.

First stage.—It is natural to suppose that the symptoms of any disease should be expressive of impeded or disordered function of the organ in which such disease is seated; and accordingly, such is the case in the present instance. Cough is generally the earliest symptom by which tuberculous disease of the lungs is indicated; but it is for some time so slight as scarcely to deserve the appellation, consisting of little more than one or two imperfect efforts to cough. It is first observed in the morning on getting out of bed. After a longer or shorter period, it occurs occasionally during the day, especially after any exertion which hurries the breathing, and also at night on getting into bed. By degrees, the morning cough is accompanied with the expectoration of a transparent ropy fluid, resembling the saliva, and apparently originating in the posterior fauces.

Along with the cough, sometimes indeed preceding it, but much more generally occurring only after it has existed for some time, a degree of oppression or quickness of breathing is remarked on ascending stairs, or making any active exertion; and a tightness of chest or transitory pain is also frequently experienced on these occasions.

Soon after the appearance of the cough and dyspnœa, the general system begins to sympathise with the local disease. The pulse becomes quicker than natural, especially after meals and towards evening. At this period of the day there is also frequently experienced a slight degree of chilliness, followed by some heat of skin, particularly in the palms of the hands and soles of the feet, which continues during the night. When this state has continued for some time, perspiration succeeds the heat, occurring generally towards morning. Yet this febrile paroxysm is often so slight as to be overlooked by the patient, particularly its two last stages; the evening chill attracts more attention, as the sensations which accompany it are very unpleasant, but it rarely occurs without being followed by a degree of febrile heat. The sleep is now less sound and refreshing, and is occasionally disturbed during the night by cough.

While these symptoms of local disease are en-
gaging our notice, those indicating the state of the
system are no less deserving of our attention. The
aspect of the patient gives evident indications of
tuberculous cachexia : the countenance is paler than
usual, or changes colour frequently, — being at
times, more especially early in the day and after a
little fatigue, faded and expressive of languor; and
this indeed exists in a greater or less degree, the
patient being little inclined or able for exertion,
either bodily or mental. On examination at this
time the skin will also be found to have lost its
natural elastic feel, and the flesh its firmness, while
a degree of emaciation is generally evident.

These symptoms may continue for a considerable
time without any remarkable increase, varying in
degree according to the state of the weather and
the circumstances in which the patient is placed. If
they have made their first appearance in the spring,
they often diminish and may even cease as the summer advances, especially if the patient is put upon
a judicious regimen, and resides in a healthy part of
the country. The tuberculous disease is interrupted
by the amendment of the general health ,and the patient may even improve so much as to lead him and
his friends to think the danger is past; but the
following season too often undeceives them. If the
disease has shewn itself early in the winter, the
amelioration produced by the succeeding summer

is seldom so evident. Still the state of the patient may undergo great amendment, and he may gain both flesh and strength; but the cough seldom ceases entirely, and the return of cold weather, or the first attack of autumnal catarrh, brings back the symptoms with remarkable rapidity.

As the *first stage* of tuberculous consumption is generally characterised by the symptoms which have been enumerated above, it becomes a matter of great importance to ascertain the condition of the lungs with which they are associated. We have seen that cough, some dyspnœa, slight hectic fever, languor, debility, and commencing emaciation constitute the external or visible phenomena of the disease. Morbid anatomy informs us that the lungs at this period contain a greater or less quantity of tuberculous matter, which is still in what is called the state of crudity,—that is, more or less firm, of a greyish colour, and somewhat transparent, or partly of a pale yellowish colour and opaque. The pulmonary tissue and bronchial membrane in the immediate vicinity of the tuberculous deposits may have undergone no perceptible alteration, or both may present a degree of redness and increased vascularity.

Physical signs.—In the very early stage of tuberculous disease the physical signs are unfortunately often obscure; although this will depend on the quantity of tuberculous matter, and the manner in which it is deposited. If the matter be in small quantity, or diffused pretty generally through the lungs, little light will be thrown on the disease by auscultation; but when more abundant, and deposited, as it generally is, in the summit of the lungs, auscultation assists us greatly in detecting the real nature of the disease in doubtful cases. The sound elicited by percussion, when delicately performed, will often be found clearer under one clavicle than the other; the respiratory murmur, heard through the stethoscope, will be less soft, and the resonance of the voice greater, where the duller sound exists. Unless, however, there is an obvious difference between the sounds heard in the relative situations on the opposite sides, the signs afforded by auscultation are not much to be depended on at this early stage; and in many cases we have to form our opinion of the patient's condition from the local and constitutional symptoms only. In other instances, however, with the same symptoms, the physical signs afford the most unequivocal indications of the existence of pulmonary disease. The sound elicited by percussion is evidently less clear under one clavicle;* the respiration less soft and

* " In no case," says Dr. Forbes, " is the importance of percussion so frequently and strikingly evinced as in the earlier stages of phthisis. A single tap on the clavicle will often afford the means of a more certain diagnosis than weeks or even months of observation of the general symptoms."--See *Translation of Laennec*, last edit., p. 308.

easy, and the voice decidedly more resonant than under the opposite clavicle; and, even at this early period, the motions of the upper parts of the chest, carefully observed during inspiration, may often be remarked to be unequal; one side of the chest being more fully expanded during inspiration than the other. When this is the case, it will generally be found that the side least elevated is that which gives the most evident signs of the existence of tubercles. When the tuberculous matter is diffused over a large portion of the lungs, a degree of puerile respiration occasionally indicates its presence. A marked inequality in the sound of the respiration in different parts of the chest also affords strong suspicion of tuberculous disease, when such inequality cannot be otherwise accounted for.

By a careful inquiry into the state of the patient's health previously to the period now under consideration, and by attention to the various symptoms which have been enumerated, the physician who has been accustomed to trace the relation of symptoms to the morbid changes of the organ, will rarely fail to arrive at a correct opinion; and if he can avail himself of the evidence derived from the physical signs, he will have the positive assurance that his diagnosis is correct in a very large proportion of cases. Yet it often happens that a patient presenting all the indications of tuberculous disease which have just been stated, is said, and believed to be, merely *threatened* with disease of the lungs, or to have an affection of the trachea or bronchi; and it is commonly added that, ' with care, all will do well.' This arises from the habit of trusting to symptoms alone for a knowledge of disease, and of neglecting pathological anatomy, without a knowledge of which the physician is unable to connect the external phenomena of disease with the morbid condition of the organ.

Second stage.—The circumstance which has been considered as indicating the transition from the first to the second stage of phthisis is a remarkable change in the expectoration. The colourless frothy fluid, which had hitherto been expectorated, is observed to contain small specks of opaque curdly matter, of a pale yellowish colour; the proportion of which gradually increases, forming patches surrounded with the transparent portion in which it seems to float. Specks or streaks of blood are also often observed in the expectoration at this time.

With this change in the expectorated matter, the other symptoms generally increase; the cough becomes more frequent, the evening chills are more severe, the succeeding heat of skin is greater and more general, and the morning perspirations are more abundant and more regular in their recurrence. The hectic fever is now established; the pulse is frequent at all times, and the respiration hurried, even when the patient is at rest. The loss of flesh is very evident, and what remains is soft and flabby; the sense of languor and debility increases, and the patient feels himself quite unequal to the bodily and mental exertion to which he had been accustomed. The face is generally pale during the day, while a circumscribed flush of the cheek is often remarked towards evening. About this period also, if not earlier, pains, which are usually considered rheumatic, are often experienced in the side and in the vicinity of one or both shoulders. Hemoptysis is likewise a frequent occurrence, amounting in some cases merely to a slight streak in the expectoration, while in others a considerable quantity of pure unmixed blood is brought up.

These symptoms are accompanied by a corresponding change in the morbid condition of the lungs. The tuberculous deposit has undergone that process which is called *softening*,—that is, it has been softened and diluted by a secretion from the surrounding pulmonary tissue; and the change in the character of the expectoration indicates at once the softening of the tuberculous matter, and its passage into the bronchial tubes. While this process is taking place in the earlier tuberculous deposits, the pleura covering the diseased portion of lung generally becomes adherent to the costal pleura, by the effusion of lymph which is subsequently converted into cellular tissue. The extent and firmness of these adhesions are generally proportionate to the extent and duration of the tuberculous disease. The pains which are very commonly experienced in the upper and lateral parts of the chest, are, no doubt, partly the consequence of the slight pleuritic inflammation which precedes the uniting process ; and accordingly I have generally found on inquiry that they were either confined to, or more frequent on that side of the chest where the most extensive tuberculous disease was manifest.

While the tuberculous matter is being thus softened and expectorated, leaving cavities of a greater or less extent in the superior lobes, the lower portions of the lungs are gradually becoming tuberculous, the progress of the disease being usually from above downwards.

A careful examination of the chest at this period affords positive evidence of the internal mischief. The upper parts are less freely raised during inspiration than in the healthy state; and this is frequently more evident on one side than the other. The sound on percussion is dull under both clavicles; and on applying the stethoscope to the chest, a slight but peculiar crackling sound *(crepitant rhonchus)* is heard. The voice is more resonant, amounting generally to bronchophony, and distinct pectoriloquy is often heard in one or more points of the clavicular or scapular regions. All these indications are very generally more evident on one side than the other; and hence, in obscure and complicated cases, arises the advantage, and even the necessity of attending particularly to this circumstance, in order to enable us to establish our diagnosis with more certainty and precision.

The extent to which the lungs have become tuberculous in the stage of phthisis now under consideration, varies remarkably in different cases, without a corresponding difference in the severity or duration of the symptoms. Two patients having symptoms exactly similar, may, on examination of their chests, present a very striking difference in the extent of the pulmonary disease; hence, by trusting to the symptoms alone, without having a due regard to the physical signs, we shall often be led into error in estimating this important point.

The length of time during which a patient may continue in the state which has been described, also varies greatly. In some cases a few weeks suffice to lead him to the brink of the grave, while in others many months, or even years, may pass without any remarkable increase or diminution of the symptoms, or, there is reason to believe, of the pulmonary affection. In a small proportion of cases a curative process is established, by which the tuberculous disease is partially or entirely obliterated; and if the patient's general health is maintained in a good state, there may be no future tuberculous deposit.

Third stage.—This has been termed the colliquative stage, from the copious perspirations, the frequent attacks of diarrhœa, and the abundant expectoration by which it is usually attended. With these symptoms, but more especially with the diarrhœa, the emaciation and debility generally keep pace: the cough also becomes more distressing during the night as the diseases advances, and the patient frequently suffers from pains of the chest; while his breathing is much oppressed on the slightest exertion. The feet and ancles become œdematous; the swelling at first disappearing in the course of the night.

The chest at this advanced period of the disease is found to be remarkably changed in its form; it is flat instead of being round and prominent; the shoulders are raised and brought forward, and the clavicles are unusually prominent, leaving a deep hollow space between them and the upper ribs. The sub-clavicular regions are nearly immoveable during respiration; and when the patient attempts to make a full inspiration, the upper part of the thorax, instead of expanding with the spontaneous ease peculiar to health, seems to be forcibly dragged upwards. Percussion gives a dull sound over the superior parts of the chest, although the caverns which partially occupy this part of the lungs, and the emaciated state of the parietes, may render the

D

sound less dull than in the preceding stage. The
stethoscope affords more certain signs: the respiration is obscure and in some places inaudible,
while in others it is particularly clear, but has the
character of the bronchial, or tracheal, or even
the cavernous respiration of Laennec. There is
a mucous rhonchus; coughing gives rise to a
gurgling sound *(gargouillement);* and pectoriloquy
is generally more or less distinct,—for the most
part on both sides, although more marked on one
than on the other. In this state the patient may
still linger for many weeks, or even months, reduced almost to a skeleton, and scarcely able to
move in consequence of debility and dyspnœa.

With the loss of physical strength, the energy of
the mind generally undergoes a corresponding diminution; the reasoning faculty remains, but its
powers are evidently enfeebled. Although in-
wardly conscious of his decay, the patient seldom
excludes the possibility of recovery, until at last
he becomes indifferent to his own state and to
what is passing around him, notwithstanding he
had been hitherto remarkably alive to every symptom.

During the last weeks of existence there is
generally an aphthous state of the mouth, which
is a sure forerunner of approaching dissolution:
delirium, of a mild character, likewise occurs at

intervals, although in some cases it is entirely absent. In a few instances I have observed violent delirium for several days preceding" death.

Such is the more common progress of tuberculous disease of the lungs, and such are the phenomena by which it is generally accompanied and characterised : we shall presently enter into a more full examination of the different symptoms.

It has often been stated that pulmonary consumption is a mild disease, by which the patient is imperceptibly wasted away, without pain or suffering, indulging the hope of recovery to the last. They must have witnessed but little of the disease who could give this as its general character. The miserable sensations produced by the frequent chills during the day, and by the more distressing and death-like chills which follow the copious perspirations in the night and morning ; the harassing cough and expectoration; the pains of the chest; the frequent dyspnœa, amounting often to a threatening of suffocation ; the distressing sense of sinking produced by the diarrhœa,—all increasing as the strength of the unfortunate patient fails;— and, more than these, that " contention de l'esprit," that inward struggle between hope and fear, which, whether avowed or not, is generally felt by the patient in the latter stages,—constitute a degree of suffering which, considering the protracted period of its duration, is seldom surpassed in any other disease.

ᵛ But as consumption differs remarkably in the rapidity of its progress, and the severity of its symptoms, so does it also in its mode of termination. In many cases the patient's sufferings give place to a state of tranquillity and ease during the last days of life; and he sinks gradually without a struggle. In other cases the struggle continues to the last.

SECT. II.—THE MORE MARKED VARIETIES OF PHTHISIS.

Although tuberculous consumption in all its forms has essentially the same anatomical characters and constitutional origin, it varies so remarkably in duration and external features as almost to appear a different disease. I shall therefore endeavour to describe its varieties, that they may be recognised in their earlier stages.

Five forms, differing from the ordinary course of consumption, appear worthy of particular notice; and I must be allowed to observe that such distinctions are not mere pretensions to refinement, but, on the contrary, are of great utility as regards both the diagnosis and treatment of the disease;

for each of these forms has something in its character which it is important to mark, in order to
recognize the nature of the disease at an early
period of its development.

ACUTE OR RAPID CONSUMPTION.—The usual
duration of consumption may perhaps be stated to
range from nine months to two years;* in the
present variety it frequently runs its course in three
or even two months, and occasionally in six weeks
and even less.

The acute form admits of a useful subdivision
into *two* varieties, in one of which the short
duration of the disease appears to depend chiefly
on its violence, or the activity of the morbid process;
and in the other, on the feeble powers of the constitution, which sinks under the pulmonary disease
long before it has reached the degree in which it
usually proves fatal.

The *first* variety shews itself in striking characters. All the symptoms of consumption in its
ordinary form are present in an unusual degree of
severity, and succeed each other with great rapidity. The cough increases from day to day, and
the expectoration passes through its various changes
in the course of a few weeks; the hectic fever is
violent, the morning perspirations are copious, and
diarrhœa usually contributes its share in the de-

---

* See chapter on STATISTICS OF CONSUMPTION.

struction of the patient, who sinks rapidly in the course of six or eight weeks; dying of what is popularly and expressively termed ' a galloping consumption.' M. Andral has given four examples of this form, three of which occurred in young subjects, varying in duration from twenty-one to thirty-five days.* Indeed, young persons are generally the subjects of this variety; and it frequently occurs soon after acute febrile diseases, as fever, scarlatina, measles, &c. The manner in which these diseases modify consumption I shall have occasion to show when treating of the exciting causes.

There are two ways in which this rapid progress of consumption may be explained. It often occurs in persons of a constitution so highly tuberculous, as only to require the application of some exciting cause to determine the deposition of tuberculous matter in the lungs. In other cases the short course of the disease is more apparent than real. The tuberculous disease of the lungs, though latent, has been making silent progress, until, from exposure to cold or violent exertion, an attack of catarrh, of pneumonia, or of hemoptysis is induced. after which the usual symptoms show themselves, and, owing to the extent of the tuberculous deposit, the disease proceeds in its course with unusual rapidity.

---

*¹ Archives Générales de Médecine, vol. ii. p. 205.

The accuracy of this view will be supported by minute inquiry into the history of such cases, and by the fact that they commonly occur in the members of families of a strongly marked tuberculous constitution.

The error into which this variety of acute phthisis is calculated to lead an inexperienced or careless practitioner, is that of considering and treating it as a purely inflammatory disease, and using more active measures, and giving a more favourable prognosis, than the case justifies. It is true that inflammation in some part of the respiratory organs often exists, complicating the tuberculous disease; but it requires to be treated with much more delicacy than a simple inflammation, and a very different prognosis should be given. An inquiry into the previous health of the patient and careful observation of the symptoms will alone unveil the real nature of the disease.

The *second* variety is observed chiefly in delicate young persons, and more frequently, according to my observation, in females than in males. The symptoms are often little marked; so little indeed that this variety might almost be ranked under the latent or occult form of the disease,—the real condition of the patient often escaping observation till the lungs are tuberculous to a considerable extent. But, although the symptoms are slight, they are generally sufficient to enable the attentive phy-

sician to recognize the disease, especially when
the general aspect and constitution of the patient
are taken into account. There is a slight cough
with some shortness of breathing; and the pulse
is frequent or easily rendered so by the slightest
exertion. The patient is weak, languid, and chilly,
but scarcely considers herself ill; there is no pain of
chest, no hemoptysis, and perhaps no expectoration.
Debility, being the most prominent symptom, is
often considered the cause of all the others, and even
when there are morning perspirations and progressive emaciation, the friends are scarcely alarmed:
they think that she was always short-breathed and
liable to catarrh, and that the lungs must be sound,
as the cough seems of so little consequence. Without any other remarkable symptom the patient gets
rapidly worse; the cough becomes more troublesome, and is by degrees accompanied by expectoration, in which a tinge of blood occasionally appears. The breathing is now observed to be very
quick, even when the patient is at rest;—the pulse
is rapid and feeble, and there are frequent and
often very copious morning perspirations. The
countenance alone, at this time, is very often sufficient to indicate the danger: it is generally pale
and of a leaden hue, the lips are of a blueish
colour, and the white of the eye has a peculiar
dull pearly tint; the whole features are fallen and
the countenance faded, except when lighted up by

a transient hectic flush. Under such circumstances the patient may sink with great rapidity from an attack of diarrhœa, or a fainting fit, on some slight exertion, may prove suddenly fatal.

This is a most insidious form of consumption, and requires the closest observation of the practitioner, as it is liable to be overlooked, both on account of the obscure character of the local symptoms, and the little importance attached to them by the patient's friends. Its victims are merely valetudinarians in their best state of health: their natural state is one of weakness; they are easily fatigued and even exhausted by exercise; they are oppressed by a high, and chilled by a low temperature:—they have the lymphatic constitution of the child without the power and activity of the child's circulating system, and yield to the ordinary causes of disease with remarkable facility. In such persons the transitions from their usual health to a state of tuberculous cachexia, and from this to actual tuberculous disease of the lungs, are easy and almost imperceptible.

FEBRILE CONSUMPTION.—-This form differs materially in its symptoms from the more common acute varieties which have just been noticed, as well as from the usual form of the disease;—even the morbid appearances discovered after death are somewhat peculiar. The degree of fever by which it is usually ushered in and attended during its whole course, is one of its most remarkable features, and the one from which I have ventured to denominate it *febrile consumption.*

Its attack is generally sudden, occurring in a state of apparent health, after exposure to cold, or even without any very evident cause. I say apparent health, because I believe that the disease only occurs in persons of a tuberculous diathesis,—the most marked cases which have come under my notice having occurred in families, several members of which had already fallen victims to the disease in its usual form.

It commences with shivering, followed by heat of skin, quick pulse, and the other symptoms of fever, which often continue for several days with little or no indications of pulmonary disease; in some cases putting on the characters of bilious, and in others of catarrhal fever, for either of which it may be mistaken.

Cough generally soon appears, and hurried breathing is one of the most remarkable symptoms. The cough speedily becomes more frequent, and is soon accompanied by some expectoration, which is at first colourless, afterwards assumes a yellowish or greenish hue, and is occasionally streaked with blood; but it has rarely the characters of the expectoration of the advanced stage of ordinary consumption. Pain of one or both sides frequently occurs, and occasionally there is diarrhœa. The fever, in the meanwhile, continues without abatement, and is so much out of proportion to the other symptoms of pulmonary affection, as to render the true character of the disease liable to be overlooked. In the course of from three to six or seven weeks the patient sinks.

As the case advances, its nature generally becomes more evident; but still the symptoms are often so little marked as to render it doubtful whether the disease is not acute bronchitis or pneumonia; and when either of these affections complicates the tuberculous disease, the diagnosis becomes extremely difficult. In some cases auscultation assists us materially. The upper parts of the chest often give a dull sound on percussion, although the tuberculous matter is less frequently confined to the summit of the lungs in this than in the other forms; a circumstance which constitutes one of its pathological characters. The whole of one side of the lungs and even a large portion of both appears to be attacked in some cases almost at the same time, giving rise to a dull sound on percussion, and bronchial respiration. Under such circumstances it is difficult to distinguish the disease from pneumonia. The negative symptoms assist us: we have neither the crepitant rhonchus which precedes the dull sound and bronchial respiration, nor the characteristic sputa of pneumonia. When, on the

other hand, this sudden deposition of tuberculous
matter does not take place in the pulmonary tissue,
but occurs in the minute terminations of the bronchi and in the air-cells to a great extent, the case
resembles acute bronchitis more than pneumonia.
Here again we derive assistance from the negative
symptoms : the bronchial sputa are wanting, and
the whole progress of the disease differs from that
of bronchitis ; there is also, for the most part, an
extreme rapidity of breathing, which is not observed in any other pulmonary affection. But
there are cases respecting the real nature of which
the most attentive observer, aided by all our means
of diagnosis, may be in doubt.

The morbid appearances of this form have been
well described by M. Louis* and Dr. Carswell.†
They are of two kinds: in one class of cases
they consist of that form of tubercle denominated grey granulations, deposited in great numbers in the lungs, the surrounding pulmonary
tissue being infiltrated with serosity, which, as Dr.
Carswell remarks, greatly augments the dyspnœa,
and may prove fatal by inducing asphyxia. In

---

* Recherches Anatomico-Pathologiques sur la Phthisie, p.
411, &c.

† *Cyclopædia of Practical Medicine*, article Tubercle,
vol. iv.

other cases the pulmonary tissue is completely infiltrated with tuberculous matter, a large portion of the lungs being converted into a mass of cheese-like substance. Louis considers this form of tuberculous deposit, when it exists to a considerable extent, peculiar to acute phthisis. Tuberculous cavities are found in some instances, but they are generally of small size, are only partially evacuated, and have no lining membrane, which is commonly the case in cavities of longer duration.

Notwithstanding the rapidity of febrile consumption, it is often attended with those morbid affections of other organs which accompany the disease in its usual form, such as ulceration of the intestines, larynx, and trachea, and the diseased states of the mucous membrane of the stomach and the liver; showing that it is true to the general character of phthisis, although differing from it in its external features.

The diagnosis in the early stage of this variety is often attended with difficulty. The sudden attack of fever with rapid respiration and some cough, occurring in a person of tuberculous constitution, should excite suspicion; and the continuance of the symptoms despite the remedies employed, together with the absence of those symptoms which characterise the common acute diseases of the chest, will greatly assist us. Per-

cussion and auscultation will also lend their aid in
many cases.*

Febrile phthisis appears most frequently to attack
young persons, although the subject of one of
Louis's cases was in his forty-sixth year; it also
occasionally supervenes upon the common form.
In this case the breathing becomes very difficult
and rapid; still the chest preserves its resonance,
the respiratory sound being accompanied with a
slight rhonchus. On examination after death, a
large quantity of grey granulations is found diffused
over a great part of the lungs, in addition to the
tuberculous disease existing previously to the acute
attack.

It is proper to remark that the disease which I
have described has been considered as a form of
pneumonia, the grey granulations being regarded
by Andral as the result of inflammation of the
air-cells; and on this view there will be equal
propriety in considering the rapid tuberculous infiltration of the lungs the result of inflammation in a
tuberculous subject. I do not think it of much
consequence to dispute this point. I believe that
inflammation in a tuberculous constitution may give
rise to the deposition of tuberculous matter in place

* M. Louis has made some good remarks on the diagnosis of
this form of phthisis, at page 437 of his work, already cited.

of coagulable lymph, which in healthy subjects is its natural product; and thus inflammation may be one of the immediate causes of tuberculous disease.

CHRONIC CONSUMPTION.—As opposed to the acute forms which have been noticed, the present variety may very properly be termed chronic, as it often occupies more years than the former do weeks. Bayle* and Laennec† were the first who described the nature of these protracted cases, and showed the identity of the disease, whether occupying the greater part of a long life, or proving fatal in the course of a few weeks.

Acute phthisis occurs most frequently, as has been remarked, in young subjects; the chronic form commonly at a more advanced period of life, from the fortieth year upwards; although it is occasionally met with at a much earlier age. In the former, the tubercular diathesis is generally hereditary and strongly marked, and the causes which usually call it into action speedily produce their effect. In the latter, on the contrary, the tuberculous diathesis, if hereditary, is not strong, or has been kept in check by the favourable circumstances in which the individual has been placed,—or it has been induced, in the progress

* Recherches sur la Phthisie Pulmonaire.
† Op. citat.

through life, by causes which I shall have
occasion to notice in another part of this work.
However this may be, the tuberculous disease of
the lungs at a late period of life is often slower in
its progress, and is attended with much less evident
symptoms, than at an earlier age.

The symptoms of chronic consumption are often
obscure in its early stages : the patient appears
out of health ; he is languid and less capable of
exertion than usual ; has occasionally a slight
cough, but it scarcely attracts attention ; he has
no fever, and the appetite is generally good. As
it very often occurs in persons whose occupations
give rise to dyspeptic complaints, the stomach is
the organ to which the indisposition is attributed.
The patient himself and his friends are often confirmed in this opinion by the beneficial effects of
fine weather, a visit to the country, or a summer
tour ; by means of which he recovers his looks
and flesh and strength, and the cough ceases. In
the succeeding winter the cough returns, he again
loses flesh, and his looks indicate internal disease,
while he is more than usually susceptible of the
impressions of cold. Still during the succeeding
summer his health improves. At times, however,
his disease assumes a more serious aspect : during
an attack of catarrh the cough becomes severe,
and is attended by fever and copious expectora-

tion,—symptoms which appear to threaten his life. Even from this state he may recover more than once, till the disease shall at last assume the form of a chronic catarrh, aggravated from time to time by slight exposure to cold during the winter and spring; but he may still enjoy a very tolerable share of health during the summer, and thus may continue to linger in a precarious state of existence for years, little aware of the real nature of his disease.

In this condition the person is generally able to pursue his usual avocations, though not with his wonted energy; and if they require much bodily exertion, or expose him to the inclemencies of the weather, they are often interrupted by attacks of acute catarrh, of pleurisy, or pneumonia. Under more favourable circumstances he may escape such attacks, but he is easily fatigued, his breathing is generally oppressed by active exercise, and he is rarely free from cough a week at one time: his appetite is generally good, he eats heartily, but remains thin and pale, and is equal to little exertion, bodily or mental. In short, though capable of attending to his usual duties, he performs them in a very different manner from that which was habitual to him, and yet his friends are scarcely aware that he is labouring under any local disease beyond a common chronic catarrh. This state of things is not uncommon in persons living in easy

circumstances, and who are not required to expose
themselves to the vicissitudes of the weather, or to
other exciting causes of disease. They are considered delicate; they find it necessary to take
care of themselves; but the nature of their ailments
frequently remains long unsuspected. The cough
is little thought of, because it does not increase
and gives very slight trouble, and even abates so
much during the summer as to be scarcely remarked : the breathing is short, but the dyspnœa
has come on so slowly as to deceive the patient,
who is hardly aware that it is a new complaint,
and thinks that he was always short-breathed.
Invalids of this description are rarely free from
dyspepsia in a greater or less degree ; they are
liable to an increase of the catarrhal symptoms
from slight exposure to cold, and are frequently
subject to attacks of diarrhœa, their recovery from
which is often tedious and protracted.

An examination of the chest under the circumstances which have just been noticed, will generally leave no doubt of the existence of tuberculous
disease of the lungs. The respiratory movement
of the upper part of the chest will be found to be
much more limited than natural, especially when
the patient makes a full inspiration. One or both
of the clavicular regions will give a dull sound, and
the voice will be more resonant, and occasionally
there will even be perfect pectoriloquy. It often

happens in such cases, that not only does tuberculous disease exist, but the tuberculous matter has
become softened and been expectorated, leaving
cavities in the summit of the lung, some of which
have been emptied of their contents, and are either
in the progress of cure or actually cicatrized.

I have already observed that such a patient may
live for many years, if his habits are temperate
and regular, and if he avoids exposure to causes
capable of inducing inflammatory affections of the
lungs. But even with these precautionary measures,
his state is very precarious; the lungs are already
partially diseased, their capacity is diminished, and
they are consequently far more liable to congestion
and to take on diseased action. An attack of bronchitis or of pneumonia, which in a healthy condition
of the lungs would have terminated favourably, often
proves speedily fatal, or leaves the patient in a
state of great debility, during which the tuberculous disease makes more rapid progress; and
he soon sinks with all the symptoms of well-
marked consumption,—yet, even under all the
circumstances which have been stated, this is not
unfrequently attributed, both by the patient and
his attendants, to the inflammatory attack, which
was merely a superadded and accidental occurrence.
The same effect will often be produced by a severe
attack of rheumatism, or fever, or any other disease
accompanied with fever, or which leaves the patient

in a debilitated state. The influenza which prevailed in this country in the summer of 1832, and
still more severely and generally in the spring of
1833, proved fatal to many such invalids, either
during its attack, or in consequence of the debility
which it induced. To persons labouring under the
earlier stages of tuberculous disease, the same
epidemic proved equally, though not so speedily
fatal; and in such patients its origin was, with
greater appearance of truth, attributed to the
influenza.

We can only account for the slow progress of
tuberculous disease of the lungs by the supposition
that the constitutional disposition to such an affection
has been slowly induced, and has never acquired
the pervading influence of hereditary disease. This
view is supported by the fact that such protracted
cases are most frequently observed in the upper
ranks of society, where the comforts of life can be
commanded, and any deviation from ordinary health
occasioned by occupations injurious to it can be
counteracted from time to time by country air and
relaxation. On the other hand, the labouring
classes are much more rarely affected by this chronic
form of consumption: the disease often occurs late
in life among them, but its progress is more rapid,
and more closely resembles its course at an earlier
age; although in females and some men, such as
coachmen and grooms, when they are not addicted

to the use of spirits, it often exists in this chronic form for years.

After death, the lungs are found to present such a mass of disease, partly tubercles and partly the effects of inflammation, as to make it difficult to say which was the primary disease:—indeed, of its nature, little is to be learned from such examinations.

This chronic variety of consumption deserves the particular attention of the physician:—first, because it is liable to be overlooked till it has made considerable progress, and the opportunity of arresting it may be lost; and, secondly, because medicine often accomplishes much more in this form than in those which are more rapid in their course. Indeed, in many of these chronic cases I believe the progress of the pulmonary affection may be often checked, and not only the patient's life prolonged, but his health materially improved. Time is given for the adoption of such measures as are calculated to amend the general health, and even to remove, or at least to check the tuberculous cachexia, and other derangements which increase the local disease:—I allude more particularly to irritation of the digestive organs, and to congestion of the liver and abdominal viscera generally,—pathological conditions which have an important share in the production of the disease, as will be shewn in the proper place.

LATENT CONSUMPTION.—The presence of tu-

berculous matter in the lungs gives rise, in a
large proportion of cases, to those symptoms which
have been already enumerated ; there are, however, instances in which this morbid product may
exist in the lungs for a long time, and even to
a considerable extent, without occasioning any local
symptoms indicative of its presence, such as cough,
expectoration, or hemoptysis, but nevertheless si-
lently effecting its work of destruction. To cases
of this kind the term *latent* has been applied.

Of one hundred and twelve cases recorded by
Louis, eight were latent ; a smaller proportion,
perhaps, than generally occurs. From the history
of these cases, and an attentive and minute examination after death, not only of the lungs but
of all the other organs, Louis entertained no doubt
of the existence of tubercles during a period varying from six months to two years in different cases,
previously to their presence being indicated by
cough, the most common local symptom. This perfectly corresponds with my own observation. In re-
tracing the history of some cases of consumption, I
have obtained satisfactory evidence that tuberculous
disease had commenced in the lungs from one to two
years or longer before it was properly attended
to, or its nature understood.

As far as my own observation enables me to
decide, I think that latent phthisis is most frequent after the middle period of life, but no age is
exempt from it.

Latent consumption presents itself in two different forms. In one, we have constitutional symptoms, such as fever, night-sweats, emaciation, diarrhœa, &c. without any local indications of the pulmonary disease; or if these be present, they are so slight as to pass unnoticed. The other form is still more important, because it is more insidious, being attended neither by constitutional nor local symptoms, until the tuberculous disease has made considerable progress: it, therefore, claims our closest attention; because, from the slowness of its course and the more limited extent of the tuberculous disease, we may possibly be able in many cases to check its further extension, if not to arrest its progress en- tirely, should we detect it at an early stage.

When constitutional symptoms, such as fever and emaciation, occur, the suspicion of the practitioner ought to be awakened, as they cannot exist unless some local affection is present; and by an accurate examination of the chest, he will most probably ascertain that the lungs are the seat of the disease. There is much more difficulty in the detection of cases unaccompanied by marked constitutional or local symptoms, and accordingly they often remain undiscovered until they arrive at an advanced stage. Yet, I cannot easily believe that an attentive observer will not see, in the aspect of his patient, sufficient indications of the existence of the tuberculous diathesis to arouse suspicion, and

lead him to inquire minutely into the condition of
the respiratory organs, the most frequent seat of
tuberculous deposits. By instituting a proper inquiry, and by a careful examination of the chest,
he will seldom fail to detect the real nature of the
patient's state: but it is the misfortune of many
such patients that they do not complain, or give
the physician an opportunity of discovering their
disease, until it is far advanced. They feel themselves out of health, are weaker, perhaps thinner
than usual, they have less energy of mind and less
bodily strength ; still they are unable to specify
any particular ailment: they rally from time to
time, and often go on in this way till their looks fix
the attention and excite the fears of their friends,
by whom they are at last persuaded to have professional advice.

The physician will often find that his opinion is
asked in such cases at a very critical period, both
for the patient and his own character. If, from
the fear of giving alarm, from carelessness in his
examination, or ignorance of the patient's real
condition, he does not form a correct diagnosis,
or adopt effectual measures to restore the general
health, to prevent tuberculous disease if it has not
already shown itself, or to check its progress if it
has already taken place, the patient is irrecoverably
lost. In a large proportion of cases, the result, no
doubt, will be fatal, in spite of all that human art

is capable of effecting; but there are many instances where the further progress of the disease
might be stayed and life prolonged for a considerable time, and others where the usual term of existence will not be much abridged, provided the patient adheres to a proper regimen. I am acquainted
with some striking examples of persons now living,
a considerable portion of whose lungs is incapable
of performing its functions, and yet with care they
enjoy a reasonable share of health. Under such
circumstances lives of great importance to their
families and to society may be preserved. Indeed,
I am satisfied that there are far more individuals in this state than is generally believed;
and it is well known that tubercles are frequently
found after death in the lungs of persons in whom
they had not even been suspected. I venture,
however, to express a firm belief that the disease
would be more frequently detected in its early
stages, and many valuable lives saved, by a due
attention to the indications of tuberculous cachexia
which present themselves in such patients.

Tuberculous disease is rendered latent, or is at
least masked by peculiar conditions of the system,
or by the presence of other diseases. Pregnancy
appears to retard if not to suspend its progress,
and it is frequently observed that it advances with
great rapidity immediately after parturition. The
catamenia generally cease when the disease has

made some progress; although in a few rare cases
they continue. An attack of mania in a phthisical
patient is occasionally followed by a suspension of
the pulmonary disease; but this rarely fails to carry
him off ultimately, whether the attack of mania has
ceased or not. The complication of dyspepsia with
tuberculous disease is not an infrequent cause of
the latter being overlooked, the dyspeptic symptoms
being more evident than the phthisical. The aspect
of the patient in such cases is pale and unhealthy;
he gets thinner and weaker; the food which he
takes affords him neither nourishment nor strength;
and yet he has no evident ailment but what is
referable to the deranged state of the digestive
organs. There may be no cough, no fever nor
expectoration to excite fears for his safety;
while at the same time tuberculous disease of
the lungs is gradually extending in these organs.
This is the form of the disease which has been
termed *dyspeptic phthisis;* a term which I consider
decidedly objectionable if used to designate a species of phthisis differing from the tuberculous;
because, however prominent may be the dyspeptic
symptoms, and however obscure the tuberculous
disease of the lungs, the latter is the cause of
death. While I admit to the fullest extent the
necessity of attending to the state of the digestive organs, I must object to the pathological view
which limits the attention of the practitioner to the

dyspeptic or hepatic affections, neglecting other and
equally essential parts of the treatment. I do not
know such a disease as dyspeptic phthisis as constituting a particular species; but I am well acquainted with the chronic form of tuberculous
consumption which is long preceded and accompanied by dyspeptic symptoms. Indeed, tuberculous
consumption rarely occurs in the middle periods of
life without this complication; but the deranged
condition of the digestive organs is, in these cases,
very often a mere consequence of a long pre-
existing state of venous congestion of the abdominal viscera; and which, if not corrected by
more efficient measures than those generally adopted
to relieve the dyspeptic symptoms, may terminate
in pulmonary consumption.*

The profession is highly indebted to Dr. Philip
for directing its attention to the congestive state of
the hepatic system, and pointing out some of the
most effectual means of obviating it; but I cannot
admit that his dyspeptic phthisis differs in its nature
from tuberculous consumption.

Diabetes occasionally complicates phthisis, the
symptoms of the latter being suspended for a time
by the influence of the former. Dr. Bardsley has

* See remarks on Strumous Dyspepsia, p. 16, &c.

particularly remarked the connection of tuberculous disease of the lungs with diabetes.*

Diarrhœa is another disease which sometimes disguises phthisis, and its effects in suspending all the usual symptoms of the pulmonary affection are often remarkable. I have known more than one example of extensive tuberculous disease of the lungs being detected on dissection, when the cause of death has been looked for in the intestines. It is true that these were cases in which the early history of the disease was neglected, but they serve at least to show the power of diarrhœa in masking extensive affections of the lungs. It is enough, however, that such facts should be known, in order that the younger members of the profession may be prevented from falling into the error of overlooking the disease of most importance, and of mistaking for the chief and primary affection, that which is only secondary both in occurrence and in consequence.

CONSUMPTION IN INFANCY AND CHILDHOOD. Since morbid anatomy has been more sedulously cultivated, tuberculous disease has been found a more frequent cause of death in childhood, and even in infancy, than was formerly imagined. In

* See his excellent article on DIABETES, *Cyclopædia of Practical Medicine,* vol. i.

France, where the extent and constitution of their hospital establishments have enabled the medical officers to investigate the morbid anatomy of disease upon a large scale, the tuberculous affections of children have of late occupied particular attention, and much valuable information has been collected on the subject. Dr. Guersent, one of the physicians to the ' Hôpital des Enfans Malades,' (an institution appropriated to the treatment of patients between the ages of one and sixteen years,) states, as the result of his observations, that five-sixths of those who die in that establishment are more or less tuberculous.*

Consumption at this early period of life differs somewhat from the disease in adults, both in its symptoms and the site of the tuberculous deposit. The cough is very often of a character different from that which accompanies consumption in persons of mature age ; it frequently occurs in paroxysms resembling those of hooping-cough, and is rarely attended with expectoration till a late period of the disease, and as the matter is frequently swallowed, we are deprived of the light which the characters of the expectoration might throw upon the nature of the disease. Hemoptysis is a rare occurrence ; at least, I do not

* *Le Blond,* Sur une espèce de phthisie particulière aux enfans. Paris, 1824.

recollect to have met with any case in which it was present. The hectic fever is likewise less perfectly formed, and the perspirations are generally less abundant than in the adult.

The disease, however, if we attend to the other symptoms, is not usually difficult of detection:—the tuberculous aspect of the child, the rapid pulse and breathing, the frequent cough, and the gradually increasing emaciation, commonly afford sufficient evidence of its nature. Consumption in children is often preceded or accompanied by considerable derangement of the digestive organs; the abdomen is tumid, the bowels are irregular, at one time constipated, and affected by diarrhœa at another;—the evacuations in either case are generally of a pale, unnatural colour. This deranged state of the functions of the abdominal viscera has led to the belief that the mesenteric glands were the chief seat of tuberculous disease; whereas in reality the bronchial glands and lungs are most commonly affected. It is true that the mesenteric glands become tuberculous more frequently in infancy and childhood than at a later period of life, but by no means so generally, nor to such an extent, as is supposed.

The disease often commences in the bronchial glands, occasionally proving fatal without affecting the lungs or any other organ; and hence it has been denominated bronchial phthisis (phthisie bron-

*chique);** and, if the term phthisis be confined to
the disease arising from tubercles, the name is unexceptionable. This form is almost peculiar to
childhood; at least it is much more frequent
at this period of life, and it is at this age only
that tuberculous disease is confined to the bronchial
glands.

M. Andral, in noticing the greater frequency of
tuberculous disease of the bronchial glands in
children than in adults, observes that this is
in accordance with the affections of the other lymphatic glands. The bronchial membrane in the
neighbourhood of the diseased glands was, for the
most part, found by this physician in a state of
inflammation, just as is frequently remarked in the
intestines of children when the mesenteric glands
are tuberculous. But although M. Andral generally found the bronchial membrane red in the
vicinity of these glands, it was not invariably so :
in some instances they were found in a tuberculous
state where there were neither symptoms of catarrh
during life, nor the least trace of inflammation,
old or recent, after death.† Still the connexion of
inflammation in the mucous membrane of the intestinal canal and bronchi with tuberculous disease of
the neighbouring glands, seems more intimate in
early life than after puberty.

---

* *Le Blond,* Op. cit.   † Clinique Médicale, t. ii. pp. 254-55.

The symptoms which indicate the presence of
tuberculous disease in the bronchial glands are
generally obscure for some time; hence they may
be tuberculous without being detected, as it is
not until they acquire a considerable size, and irritate or compress the bronchi mechanically, that the
local symptoms become evident. The child coughs,
is short-breathed, very liable to catarrh, and occasionally points to the upper part of the chest as the
seat of uneasiness. But the same symptoms may
be produced by common catarrh or pulmonary
tubercles. When the diseased state of these glands
is further advanced, the nature of the case is more
easily detected. If cough, hectic fever, and emaciation occur in a child, and a careful examination
discovers tuberculous disease neither in the lungs
nor in the mesenteric glands, we may feel tolerably
certain of its existence in the bronchial glands.
" Judging from my own experience," says Dr. Carswell, "and from the fact already noticed, viz. the great
frequency of tuberculous disease of the bronchial
glands in children, and particularly at the origin
of the bronchi, I should not hesitate to give it as
my opinion, that, if a patient, of from four to
ten years of age, were affected with considerable
difficulty of breathing, without any lesion of the
lungs or other obvious cause capable of giving rise
to this modification of the function of respiration,
such a patient had tuberculous disease of the bron-

chial glands with compression of the bronchi near the bifurcation of the trachea." " A diminution in the capacity of the bronchi is not unfrequently produced by the presence of tuberculous matter situated external to these tubes. I have met with several examples in children, of compression of the large bronchi, which was the obvious cause of the difficult breathing observed during life. The tuberculous enlargement of the bronchial glands has appeared to me the sole cause of this change in the capacity of the large bronchi, and in some cases the difficulty of breathing which they occasion by compressing one or both divisions of the trachea, is very great. Such cases puzzle the physician extremely; for a clear sound may be elicited by percussion from every part of the chest, and by means of the stethoscope the respiratory murmur may be distinctly heard, although feeble, throughout the whole of both lungs."* In some cases these glands are so much enlarged as to fill up a great portion of the posterior mediastinum, and even to produce a swelling by the side of the trachea, which is visible externally; but this is rare.

Tuberculous disease, however, is not in general long limited to the bronchial glands; other organs, especially the lungs, become tuberculous, and the symptoms are then of course complicated.

* Op. citat.

Still the disease may prove fatal while confined to these glands.

It is not quite a matter of indifference whether the seat of the tuberculous disease be the bronchial glands or the lungs. In the former situation the progress of the disease is slower, continuing in some cases for years, during which the little patient may enjoy pretty good health; the disease, being seated in organs much less essential to life than the lungs, interferes less with the general functions of health, and time is afforded for the correction of the constitutional disorder.

The termination is various. That the tuberculous matter deposited in the bronchial glands may be removed by absorption, as occurs in the lymphatic glands of the neck, we have every reason to believe; but this is, no doubt, the less frequent termination. Another mode of cure is that by which the softened tuberculous gland empties itself into the bronchial tube with which it is in contact, in consequence of ulcerative absorption of the walls of the tube, as is shown in Dr. Carswell's illustrations.* The matter having passed into the bronchial tube, the cavity in which it was contained gradually contracts till it is obliterated; and the cure, as far as this gland is concerned, is complete.

---

* Illustrations of the Elementary Forms of Disease.— TUBERCLE.

The less frequent cure is that in which a portion of the gland, or rather of the tuberculous matter, remains in a cretaceous state.

The prognosis of this form of consumption must always be doubtful, inasmuch as it depends on circumstances which we are generally unable to ascertain, namely, the extent to which the bronchial glands are diseased, and whether tuberculous matter is at the same time deposited in the lungs: the degree of tuberculous cachexia under which the child labours, and the character of the constitution generally, will also materially influence our opinion respecting the ultimate result of the case. The prognosis, however, will be more favourable than when the disease exists in the lungs.

CHAPTER III.

PARTICULAR SYMPTOMS AND SIGNS OF CONSUMPTION.

HAVING described the usual course of consumption and the various forms which it occasionally assumes, I shall now take a more minute survey of the particular symptoms. To have done this while describing the progress of the disease would have interrupted and weakened the general narrative: I have thought it better, therefore, at the risk of some repetition, to devote a particular chapter to an examination of the most important symptoms and the physical signs, with the view, more especially, of determining the *Diagnosis* of the disease in its different stages.

SECT. I.—SYMPTOMS.

We have already seen that the symptoms vary greatly in different cases, as regards the time of their appearance, the order of their succession, and the degree of their severity. In analysing our observations more closely, we shall also find that there is scarcely one, even of the leading symptoms, which may not be absent; and it has been stated that instances have occurred in which tuberculous disease has proved fatal almost without any local symptoms. This, however, is by no means in accordance with my own experience; certainly I have never met with such a case, nor can I easily believe that tuberculous disease of the lungs should run its course without affording sufficient indications of its existence. If cough and expectoration be wanting, we shall find hurried breathing; and if regular hectic be absent, there will still be the rapid pulse, or the frequent chills, the night perspiration, or diarrhœa, and emaciation: more or fewer of these symptoms are always present, and, together with the peculiar cachectic character of the countenance, enable us to detect the real nature and seat of the disease. There will at least be found enough, I believe, in the most obscure cases, to excite the suspicions of the observing practitioner; and when these are once aroused, the *physical signs*, which diseases of the lungs always afford, will soon satisfy him respecting the real nature of the malady.

It is a matter of great importance to know the commencement of tuberculous disease of the lungs by its external manifestations, and to distinguish it from the other diseases with which it is liable to be

confounded; since, in a very large proportion of
cases, it is only in the early stage that we can hope
to effect a cure, or even to arrest its further
progress. The symptoms by which the first
existence of pulmonary tubercle is characterised,
are unfortunately very equivocal; added to which,
we are often baffled in our inquiry by the unwil-
lingness of the patient and the friends to aid us.
Yet, notwithstanding the doubtful character of the
early symptoms, and the obstacles which often
present themselves to us in our investigations, I
fear it is more frequently attributable to our own
neglect in seeking for information respecting the
past and present condition of the patient's health,
and to our inattention to the existing indications,
than to the real obscurity of the case, that tuberculous disease is allowed to pass undetected in
its early stages.

When we are consulted by a person whose condition induces us to suspect the existence of tubercles, our examination should be full and complete.
The aspect of the patient must not be overlooked:
the past health and occupations, the previous
diseases, and the family predisposition also (when
possible), should be ascertained; while the condition of the more important functions, and above
all that of the respiratory organs, should be investigated by all the diagnostic means in our power.
The form and motions of the chest, the sounds

elicited by percussion, and those produced by the
ingress and egress of air during respiration, speech,
and cough, must all be called to our aid to enable
us to estimate the value of particular symptoms,
—or, in the absence of these, to form a probable
opinion of the state of the lungs.

In the early period of tuberculous disease there
is no one local sign or symptom to be depended
upon ; but by a careful analysis of the whole of
them, and by availing ourselves also of the negative
symptoms, as regards other pulmonary diseases
with which consumption is liable to be confounded,
we shall rarely err in forming a correct diagnosis
at a very early stage of phthisis.

COUGH.—Cough is generally the earliest indication of pulmonary irritation, and the first circumstance which excites the attention of the patient or
his relatives. During the first weeks or months, it
is usually slight, occurring chiefly, and perhaps
only, in the morning : it is often overlooked
by the patient, or it appears to arise from irritation in the region of the larynx, and to be of no
consequence; he rarely suspects that it can have
any connection with the state of the lungs. Its
continuance in this trifling degree for weeks or
even months, without any expectoration, is a circumstance in the history of the tuberculous cough which
deserves particular attention. By degrees, it occurs
occasionally during the day, especially after any

exertion, such as running up stairs, speaking or
reading aloud for some time, or laughing; and
after a longer or shorter time it is attended with the
expectoration of a transparent frothy fluid resembling saliva, which at first appears to come from
the fauces.

In general, as the pulmonary disease advances,
the cough is found to increase, being usually in proportion to the rapidity of its course.   In some cases,
however, it is very slight through the whole disease, and, in a few rare instances, it has only
appeared a few days before death, even in cases
where tuberculous excavations of the lungs existed
to a considerable extent.   Louis gives two well-
marked examples of this.*   Now, if cough could
be absent under such circumstances until within
a few days of death, it is reasonable to admit
that it might be so altogether; and cases are
on record in which it has never occurred.   " It
is not sufficiently known," says Portal, " that the
disease can exist without the slghtest cough : the
lungs of consumptive patients have even been destroyed by suppuration, without their having experienced the least degree of cough."†   Lieutaud,
Morgagni, and others, have mentioned similar

---

* See, also, *Andral*, Clinique Médicale, tom. ii. ob. xi.

† Observations sur la Nature et le Traitement de la Phthisie
Pulmonaire, vol. ii. p. 123.   Paris, 1809.

cases.* I have never met with a case in which the cough was entirely absent, but have known it so slight as to fail to attract the attention of a very nervous patient, and of his watchful friends.

In the progress of chronic phthisis, even during the existence of tuberculous excavations, it occasionally happens that, when the patient is placed in favourable circumstances, both the cough and expectoration disappear for weeks, but usually return upon the slightest attack of catarrh.

As the disease advances, the cough occurs at all times, and without any evident cause of excitement, but is most frequent in the mornings and evenings : the rest by night is often broken by it, and by day it frequently brings on pain of the chest, and occasionally vomiting. In the latter stages it is followed by a degree of breathlessness amounting in some cases to a sense of suffocation, which is very distressing. Such are the usual characters of the cough which attends tuberculous disease of the lungs in its various stages, when not complicated with other morbid states of those organs. To these may be added another circumstance deserving notice, — no cause can in general be assigned for its first occurrence. While

* Hist. Anat. Med., lib. ii. ob. 384. De Sed. et Caus. Morb. Epist. xix.

cough is one of the earliest indications of pulmonary tubercle, it is among the most constant attendants during its progress,—a symptom most
harassing to the patient and most distressing to the
friends.

Catarrhal cough.—This is very liable to be confounded with the tuberculous cough, although in
general they may be distinguished. The cough of
catarrh is characterised by the following circumstances : — its first attack is well marked, and
can on most occasions be traced to exposure to a
cold or damp atmosphere, to checked perspiration,
or to a similar cause : it is deep, implicating the
whole respiratory muscles, and is attended by
general soreness of the chest, frontal headach,
and other symptoms of catarrh. The difference
in the expectoration which. attends these coughs
is equally well marked. The catarrhal cough,
although at first dry and hoarse, is soon accompanied with expectoration, which is at first colourless, but shortly becomes opaque, yellowish, and
even assumes a muco-purulent character. From
this time the cough and expectoration generally
diminish, and under ordinary circumstances soon
cease.

Such are the characters and usual progress of the
cough of acute catarrh ; but when the disease
assumes the chronic form,—the principal and almost

only remaining symptom being cough with more or less expectoration,—the distinction is attended with greater difficulty : yet still both the cough and the expectoration may in general be recognised in cases of pure catarrh :—it is from their complication that the difficulty arises.

When, from the continuance of the cough or from its doubtful character, we suspect some cause beyond catarrh, we should inquire carefully into the patient's state before its occurrence. If a slight morning cough, or shortness of breathing existed, or hemoptysis had occurred previously to the attack of catarrh, there are strong grounds to suspect that the continuance of the symptoms is partly dependent on tuberculous disease, more especially if the patient is young. At a more advanced period of life, we often meet with dyspnœa and a morning cough, the consequence of the dry, or pituitous catarrh, complicated frequently with emphysema of the lung.

Gastric cough.—The cough which is next in importance, in a diagnostic point of view, is that which has not inaptly been termed the *stomach cough*. Gastric irritation is frequently attended with cough, not unlike that which accompanies the early stage of tuberculous disease. A little attention, however, will enable us to discriminate them. In general, the cough which attends gastric irritation is louder and harder than the phthisical, and frequently comes on in paroxysms : the source

of irritation is felt deep in the epigastric region;
and the irritated state of the stomach is generally
rendered manifest by other symptoms. The tongue
is red at the point and edges, generally furred in
the centre, and often dry on waking in the morning; there are thirst, some quickness and a contracted state of the pulse; the extremities are cold
during the day, and a preternatural heat of the
hands and feet often prevails during the night;
the bowels are generally costive, and the urine is
high-coloured. These symptoms are frequently accompanied by frontal headach, especially in the
evening, and by an irritability of temper unusual
to the patient. If he is accustomed to mental occupations, he finds himself less disposed and less
able to exert his mind. The expression of his
countenance also changes remarkably,—he becomes
pale and sallow, and his features are fallen: he
has the look of ill-health; he feels unwell, and
yet, on being questioned, he cannot fix upon any
local complaint. This state often continues for a
long period, and in many cases without much loss
of appetite,—a circumstance which tends to deceive the patient respecting the seat and nature of
the malady.

An attentive investigation will generally satisfy
us that the disease is seated in the digestive organs,
and we shall find that the cough and other symptoms will gradually yield to proper treatment,

and the health will be frequently restored in a very short time, especially if the patient is young. A gentle antiphlogistic treatment, and a strict adherence to a mild diet, will soon show the nature of the disease, by the marked and speedy relief which they afford ; and, in truth, will be at once the best test of the accuracy of our diagnosis and the soundness of our pathological views as to the cause of the cough. Even when gastric irritation is complicated with incipient consumption, (a very frequent occurrence,) our treatment must be directed in the first instance to the cure of the former, as the surest means of enabling us to arrive at a correct knowledge of the patient's condition.

There is another form of cough which properly belongs to the stomach, as it originates in, and is kept up by, a deranged state of that organ. This cough occurs later in life. It is accompanied by a considerable expectoration of tenacious mucus, which, from its occurring chiefly in the morning, has received the name of " morning phlegm." It is generally the consequence of too free living, and accompanies the last ten or fifteen years of the gourmand's life : it is easily distinguished from the tuberculous cough.

Both these stomach coughs deserve attention, not only on their own account, but more especially when they occur in a tuberculous constitution. The

first form of the gastric irritation, when of long
duration, greatly favours the formation of the tuberculous diathesis ; and may thus prove fatal from
its nature being mistaken and its treatment mis-
directed. The second occasionally masks tuberculous disease occurring at a more advanced period
of life.

Abdominal cough.—Irritation of the liver and
duodenum, intestinal worms, and irritation of the
uterus often give rise to cough. The cough which is
present in chlorotic patients, and which is probably
dependent on functional derangement of the uterus,
may in general be easily distinguished from the
phthisical cough, by the other symptoms with which
it is associated, and by the facility with which it
yields to a mode of treatment which would have
little effect in relieving the latter. It must be kept
in mind, however, that young females of a tuberculous constitution are the persons most liable to
chlorosis, and on this account their cough must
not be treated too lightly, nor a prognosis given
without circumspection.*

Nervous cough.—This is the term applied to
another form of cough which has been confounded with the tuberculous ; but its character, the
periods at which it occurs, its mode of attack and

---

* *De Haen* has noticed the various abdominal diseases which
produce cough. Vid. Rat. Medendi, lib. iii. p. 375.

disappearance, all differ from those of the tuberculous cough. The nervous cough occurs at irregular
times throughout the day, and whatever agitates or
affects the patient's mind is liable to bring it on. It
has a peculiarly sharp, barking sound, is repeated
in quick succession at short intervals, and often
continues an hour without any intermission. It
occurs most frequently in young nervous females,
and is generally accompanied with other indications
of nervous irritability, and not unfrequently with
evident hysteria, of which indeed it may in
general be considered a modification. In all
its essential characters, therefore, the nervous
differs from the consumptive cough ; and in pure
cases there is little danger of their being confounded. In truth, all these coughs have their own
peculiar characters, by means of which they may,
with ordinary attention, be readily distinguished
when they are not complicated with each other. It
is from their existence in the same individual that
the difficulty of discrimination arises, and such
combinations frequently occur.

The tuberculous cough is very often complicated
with the catarrhal. The former often exists for
some time without attracting attention, when an
attack of catarrh occurs, which masks the consumptive cough that preceded it ; and after the
catarrh has passed through the acute stage, a cough
remains which is neither catarrhal nor tuberculous,

but partakes of the characters of both; and it is only by careful observation that we are enabled to determine its real nature. Indeed the characters of the cough will not always enable us to do so. All the other circumstances of the patient,—his previous health, his present state and appearance, his hereditary predisposition, &c., must be considered; as they will aid us in determining the nature of the affection,—whether it be an unmixed chronic irritation of the bronchial membrane, or an irritation kept up by tubercles. If tubercles are present, we shall find by attentive observation that the cough varies in its character, being at times more allied to the tuberculous, and at others to the catarrhal, especially on exposure to a cold or humid atmosphere.

The stomach and hepatic cough may, in like manner, occur in tuberculous subjects; and we may for some time be unable to ascertain the seat of the irritation which produces it. A proper regimen and such means as are known to relieve gastric irritation, and hepatic congestion, generally produce a decided effect on the cough arising from these causes.

Again, the tuberculous cough of young hysterical or nervous females is often greatly modified; sometimes assuming the nervous character to such a degree as to pass entirely for that. Both the patient and her relatives are generally

willing to believe that the cough is purely nervous,
and are anxious to impress upon the mind of the
practitioner that it is so. Mistakes of this kind have
occurred ; we must not therefore allow ourselves to
be deceived by the too favourable report of friends,
in their anxiety to make the case appear what they
wish it to be ; nor rest satisfied with the cough
which we may hear at a forenoon visit; but inquire into its character when the patient rises
in the morning and retires to rest at night, also
during exertion, and in a state of perfect quiet.
Whenever doubt exists, it is ill-judged kindness to
omit a full investigation of the case, from fear of
alarming the patient or the friends.

An examination of the chest, when performed
with caution and judgment, will be more easily
submitted to by the patient, and prove far more
satisfactory at this period of the disease, than when
it is farther advanced; at any rate, if mischief
exists, it cannot be too soon detected, even at the
risk of exciting alarm. After such an investigation
the physician can speak with decision respecting
the measures which it is necessary to adopt; and
in place of the lukewarm and vacillating directions which are too often given, he can impress
with firmness upon the minds of the relatives
the necessity of a strict adherence to such
a mode of treatment, and such prophylactic mea-

sures, as the case may require and the circumstances of the patient admit: I say prophylactic
treatment, because I am supposing the case to be
in that stage in which the chief objects of treatment are to correct the tuberculous diathesis by
general measures, and to prevent a further deposit of
tuberculous matter by avoiding those causes which
are known to irritate the respiratory organs.

DYSPNŒA.—This symptom, although never wanting, varies greatly in the degree of its intensity in
different cases. In some instances it occurs early
in the disease, being among the first circumstances
which attract the patient's attention; and it is one
of the most constant and remarkable symptoms in
the *febrile* form of the disease. When the tuberculous disease makes slow progress, dyspnœa is
little felt; and in persons who, from their quiet
mode of living, use little exercise, it is scarcely
noticed even when the frequency of the respiration
is nearly doubled. In such cases the oppression in
breathing experienced during exertion is very often
attributed to debility. Indeed, it is by no means
uncommon to find the patient unwilling to admit
the existence of dyspnœa until minutely questioned.
Consumptive patients are often jealous of being
interrogated respecting any symptom connected
with pulmonary disease; and they occasionally
conceal symptoms from the physician, who, if he

desires to arrive at the truth, must put his questions with great caution, and without appearing to attach much importance to them.

We shall not, I believe, err far in stating that the degree of dyspnœa or hurried respiration (for I class both under the same head) will generally be found proportionate to the extent of the tuberculous disease of the lungs and to the rapidity of its progress. Of a hundred and twenty-three cases reported by M. Louis, three only presented examples of severe dyspnœa; and a careful examination of the whole contents of the thorax after death, detected nothing by which to explain it. Congestion of the lungs frequently occurs in persons of a tuberculous constitution, both before and after the formation of tubercles, and may be one cause of dyspnœa; and hence we frequently find that an attack of hemoptysis, or venesection employed to subdue it, relieves both the cough and dyspnœa for a considerable time. On the other hand, it not unfrequently happens that the origin of the difficult breathing is dated from an attack of hemoptysis: I have frequently observed this, but am unable to account for it. I here allude to the protracted dyspnœa; that which immediately succeeds the attack of hemoptysis most probably depends upon the effusion of blood into the pulmonary tissue, and the consequent compression and obliteration of the air-cells to a greater or less extent. We are not yet acquainted with all the causes of dyspnœa; one is often to be found in a feeble heart, which, by being easily oppressed, gives rise to it.

Dyspnœa, therefore, although not much to be relied on as an indication of the very early stage of consumption, should always be a subject of inquiry; and it will be found, I imagine, more frequently present than is generally believed. It is experienced chiefly during exertion, and as it differs little for some time from the oppression which in a slight degree always accompanies exertion, it seldom attracts attention. Being slow and gradual in its increase, and, like many other morbid states, unattended with pain, it is little noticed until it has become very considerable. But as tuberculous disease of the lungs cannot exist to any extent without more or less dyspnœa, the presence of this symptom together with emaciation should induce us to examine the chest with care, even were there no other indications by which consumption might be suspected.

EXPECTORATION.—When the cough has continued for some time, it becomes gradually softer, and a transparent, ropy fluid, resembling saliva, is expectorated, assuming by degrees a more stringy and tenacious character. After a longer or shorter period, varying remarkably in different cases, specks of opaque matter appear mixed with the transparent frothy fluid. These specks differ in appearance, being at one time white, at another yellow or even approaching to green, and again very frequently of an ash colour, partly sinking in water in little masses, and partly floating in it in the form of striæ.

Immediately before, or at the time of this change in its character, the expectoration is occasionally tinged with blood. As the disease advances, the transparent tenacious portion diminishes, while the opaque increases and gives a more homogeneous aspect to the expectoration, which is now of a yellowish colour, and is brought up by the cough with more ease and in more distinct masses. At a later period it is of an ash colour, and is ejected in separate, rounded, flocculent-looking masses, enveloped in the transparent ropy portion. If thrown into water at this period, some of these masses sink to the bottom; others are suspended at different depths, connected together by 'the ropy, fluid expectoration before mentioned.

The period of the disease at which this last change in the character of the expectoration takes place varies in different cases, and occasionally occurs only a few days before death. But more generally these ash-coloured, distinct masses are expectorated for many weeks or months, being accompanied with more or less of the mucous fluid in which they frequently float. Bennet mentions these ash-coloured sputa as occurring, in hopeless cases, towards their termination.* In some instances the sputa retain the yellowish puriform character, forming smooth, flat, patches; and in a still smaller proportion the semitransparent tenacious expectoration continues till within a few days of death, forming a gelatinous-looking mass, separated with difficulty from the vessel which contains it. During the last days of life the expectoration is in a more dissolved state, and sometimes of a darker hue; about this period also, and often long before, it has a very fetid odour; finally it diminishes considerably, and often disappears entirely some days previous to death.

Such are the changes generally observed in the character of the expectoration; but it is right to state that they are by no means constant. The periods in the progress of tuberculous consumption at which expectoration commences, and at which the various changes occur, differ, as we have seen, in different cases. The nature, also, of the sputa is greatly affected by accidental causes, as by catarrh and pulmonic inflammation.

Few of the symptoms have excited more attention than the expectoration, or were formerly considered of equal importance to it in distinguishing consumption from bronchial disease. Since the

---

* Theatrum Tabidorum, cap. xxiv.

nature of tubercles has been more fully demonstrated by modern pathologists, and we have become acquainted with the physical signs by which
the existence of pulmonary disease is more certainly
determined, the expectoration has been much less
regarded as a means of discriminating consumption.
Pus, which was so carefully looked for, and to re-
cognise which so many experiments were made, is
now well known to be present when only bronchial
disease exists; it does not therefore form an essential character of tuberculous expectoration. But
although no physician of the present day would
think of relying on the expectorated matter as a
test of the nature of the pulmonary affection, still
a knowledge of the characters exclusively belong-
ing to the expectoration which accompanies tuberculous disease is interesting. The transparent,
frothy, tenacious sputum, though it often indicates
the presence of tubercles, is evidently a secretion
from the bronchial membrane, and may occur independently of any tuberculous disease. The same
may be said of the yellowish-green expectoration,
which is often discharged in large quantities in
chronic catarrh, and towards the termination of
bronchitis; and there is no doubt that the greater
part of the expectoration in tuberculous diseases of
the lungs is derived from the same source.

There are two characters, however, which may
be considered peculiar to the expectoration attend-

ing tuberculous disease; the striated state of the
expectorated mass with a mixture of whitish frag-
ments in it, and the ash-coloured globular masses
which are observed in the more advanced stage of
the disease. I have never seen this last form unaccompanied by tuberculous disease; but it has
been observed by Chomel and Louis in two cases
during the last days of life, where neither tubercles
nor tuberculous excavations, nor dilated bronchi
were detected after death. The very circumstance,
however, of its having been found only in two
cases, by such accurate observers, shows how very
generally it is connected with tuberculous disease.
The different characters of the expectoration already
noticed present themselves, for the most part, as has
been before stated, in the course of pulmonary
consumption. They occurred in all the cases
described by Louis, with three exceptions, in
which the ash-coloured masses never appeared,
the expectoration continuing semi-transparent, or
of a slightly yellowish hue, to the last.

The quantity of matter expectorated varies remarkably in different cases, and is by no means
commensurate with the extent of pulmonary disease.
Occasionally the quantity is extremely small, although after death large excavations are found. On
the other hand, even in the early stages, while the
expectoration is still transparent, the quantity is
often very great, especially when the disease makes

rapid progress. In a few rare cases expectoration
has been entirely wanting; Portal says that "sometimes this purulent expectoration is wanting, although the lungs be filled with abscesses."* I have
only met with one decided case in which the absence
of expectoration continued to the last;—on examination, the lungs on one side were found converted
almost entirely into a mass of tuberculous disease,
containing numerous small tuberculous vomicæ and
one of considerable size : the upper part of the other
lung was also tuberculous, and some of the tubercles
were softened. The cough in this case was so
slight as scarcely to be remarked; but the rapid
pulse, the quick breathing, the night-sweats and
emaciation were more than sufficient to indicate the
nature of the disease, independently of auscultation,
which left no doubt on the mind :—there were,
however, circumstances in the case, which, without
the assistance of auscultation, would have thrown
a shade of obscurity on its nature. In other instances large excavations are found communicating
freely with the bronchi, although, for a considerable period before death, neither cough nor expectoration was present.†

In regard to the sources of the expectorated

---

* " Quelquefois ce crachement (pus) n'a pas lieu, quoique les
poumons soient pleins de foyers de suppuration." Op. cit.

† *Andral*, Clinique Médicale, loc. citat.

matter, it is evident that when the tubercles are still in a crude state, it must be supplied by the bronchial membrane. The air-cells and terminations of the bronchi have been demonstrated by Dr. Carswell to be the primary and chief seat of tuberculous matter; and we can easily understand how its accumulation must prove a source of irritation, and that this irritation should be first communicated to the adjacent mucous membrane. The surface of tuberculous excavations affords an additional supply of matter; the quantity from this source would appear in some cases to be great, whereas in others it is extremely small; indeed I have frequently been surprised at the small quantity of the sputa compared with the extent of the caverns.

Upon a review of the preceding facts respecting the varying characters of the expectoration, the uncertainty of its changes according to the progress of the disease, and its occasional entire absence,—it follows that much reliance is not to be placed on it, either in a negative or positive sense, as a diagnostic symptom, especially in the early stages of the disease. In conjunction with other symptoms, it has considerable value in the more advanced stages, in enabling us to ascertain the presence of tuberculous disease in obscure or complicated cases, and to mark the changes which occur in the ordinary progress of phthisis.

HEMOPTYSIS. — Hemoptysis has been long regarded as a frequent cause of consumption, from
its being often observed to precede the other symptoms. A more correct knowledge of its nature
has placed hemoptysis among the consequences of
the pathological conditions of the lungs which
precede and accompany the development and
progress of tuberculous disease. It is rarely, if
ever, a cause of phthisis. It may indeed prove a
determining cause, by the debility it induces when
very copious, or by sanguineous depletion carried
to a great extent for the purpose of suppressing it :
the effusion of blood, also, into the pulmonary tissue
may become a source of irritation, or may even form
a nidus for the primary deposit of tubercle, as
M. Andral has shewn.* But hemoptysis is in
general to be regarded as an indication of the
presence of tubercles in the lungs ; although in
some cases it may be more intimately connected
with their production.

It is certain that pulmonary hemorrhage occasionally occurs in a state of apparent health, being
the first cognizable symptom of the approaching
mischief. M. Andral relates some cases in which
he thinks he had evidence that no tubercles existed
in the lungs previously to the hemoptysis, because
there were no appreciable symptoms of their

* Path. Anat. Transl. vol. ii. p. 533.

presence; and he cannot without difficulty believe
that tubercles could exist to a degree sufficient to
give rise to hemorrhage, without being preceded by
cough or some other indication of their presence.
In such cases he considers that the blood effused
into the lungs forms a matrix for tuberculous deposits.* But to produce this effect the effusion must
take place in a tuberculous constitution, which,
indeed, this distinguished pathologist admits. He
gives a case illustrative of his views, which,
while it shows that the effused blood may be the
primary seat of tubercle, supports the opinion that
tubercles would have been formed only in a tuberculous subject:—tubercles were found in a coagulum
of blood effused into the pulmonary tissue, and in
no other part of the lungs; but the patient had
tuberculous peritonitis at the same time.†

Although, therefore, hemorrhage of the lungs
may, in a few rare cases, give rise to phthisis, even
in these few it is only to be regarded as a determining cause: it is generally to be considered
symptomatic of the existence of tubercles, and is,
in this point of view, a most important symptom.

Hemoptysis is, no doubt, occasionally idiopathic,
or at least totally unconnected with any previous
disease of the lungs. In such cases a temporary
state of plethora of the lungs most probably occurs,

---

* Loc. cit.   † Clinique Médicale, tom. ii. p. 39,

which, if not caused by local injury, is either vica-
rious of the catamenia, or produced by a plethoric
state of the system, the frequent consequence of
suppressed sanguineous discharges, such as the
hemorrhoidal flux, and epistaxis. In phthisical
patients I believe that a general plethora of the
lungs often exists, and is the determining cause
both of hemoptysis and of tubercles; and that,
in such cases, the discharge of blood from the
overloaded vessels may afford relief. Hemoptysis
is occasionally dependent on disease of the heart,
and appears sometimes to be the effect of the
violence of the cough in the advanced stage of
phthisis.

Portal remarks that those who habitually spit
blood, rarely become phthisical, and cites the following observation of Baillou: " Magnas excre-
tiones sanguinis ex pulmone minus esse periculosas
quam parvas." This remark is most probably
founded on the circumstance that idiopathic hemoptysis, connected simply with congestion of the
lungs, is generally abundant; as I have observed in
the majority of the cases of this kind which have
come under my observation. But at the same time
it must be admitted that cases of idiopathic hemoptysis are very rare, in comparison with those in
which it is connected with tuberculous disease of
the lungs. M. Louis, from careful and extensive
observations on the occurrence of hemoptysis in

different diseases, came to the conclusion, that, with
the exception of some cases in which the hemorrhage depended on external injury, or was connected with suddenly suppressed catamenia, it indicates, with a high degree of probability, the presence
of tubercles in the lungs.   My own experience is
in support of this conclusion.

The influence of sex and age in the production
of hemoptysis is not undeserving of attention.
In the practice of M. Louis it occurred more frequently in females than in males, in the proportion
of three to two.   The age of the females was most
commonly from forty to sixty-five, that is, after the
period at which the catamenia usually cease,—the
reverse, Louis remarks, of what should have occurred had the hemoptysis been an effect of amenor-
rhœa or a substitute for the suppressed catamenia.
We shall probably find an explanation of this in
the circumstance that females at this age very often
become full and plethoric, and hence more liable
to attacks of inflammation and hemorrhage than
at any other period of life.   I have remarked this
particularly in females who have been subject to
very copious catamenial discharges.   Louis observed
it to occur among men nearly in the same proportion at all ages.

The frequency of the attacks of hemoptysis was
observed by Louis to be generally in proportion to
the length of the disease; when copious, it rarely

occurred oftener than twice or thrice in the same
individual. In the whole of his cases it was present
in a greater or less degree in two-thirds ; and the
numbers in which it was copious and inconsiderable
were nearly equal. In some persons it is a frequent
symptom during the whole course of the disease ;
in others it is never present. In the phthisis of
advanced life and in young children it is rare, and
occurs generally towards the close of the disease.
Hemoptysis may appear at any stage of consumption ; in a few rare cases it is, as I have remarked, the very first circumstance which excites
alarm, occurring even before the cough. When it
preceded the other symptoms, M. Louis observed that
it came on suddenly in the midst of perfect health
and without any appreciable cause. Neither of
these remarks is quite in accordance with my observation ; I have generally found that the aspect
of the patient was by no means indicative of perfect
health, although he may not have complained ; and
I have more frequently known the hemorrhage to
succeed bodily exertion, such as running, ascending
heights, or long speaking, than when no such
evident cause had occurred. In these cases I
have observed that the hemoptysis did not appear
until some hours after the exertion. One young
man, for example, had made considerable efforts in
ascending a hill ; he returned to dinner, and was
attacked with hemoptysis while dressing : another,

after great exertion in endeavouring to catch a
horse, was affected in a similar manner a few hours
after ; and a third, after delivering a lecture in
the evening, was attacked during the night.

The quantity of blood discharged at one time
differs greatly ; in some instances it does not
exceed a single mouthful, and in others it amounts
to a pint or more. Slight hemoptysis is often
confined to the mornings : when it proves fatal,
which is generally towards the termination of the
disease, the structure of the lungs is extensively
destroyed, and several pints may be suddenly discharged. The hemorrhage, in these fatal cases,
arises, for the most part, from an opening occurring suddenly in an artery of considerable
size which has been implicated in the tuberculous disease.

As a diagnostic symptom, hemoptysis is very
important. I have already stated the very large
proportion of cases in which it has been found to
indicate tuberculous disease. Its occurrence, therefore, before or soon after the commencement of
the cough, renders the presence of tubercles highly
probable.

PAIN OF CHEST.—Acute pain rarely attends
the early stage of phthisis ; but some degree of
pain is frequently experienced in the upper parts
of the chest and shoulders, although rarely mentioned by the patient unless inquiry be made on the

subject, and then it is generally attributed to rheumatism. As the disease advances, pain is a more frequent symptom, and is generally most severe on that side in which tuberculous disease is most extensive.

I have noticed the slight pains in the clavicular regions, because in doubtful cases they would increase our suspicions of the presence of tuberculous disease; especially when other symptoms, such as the tuberculous character of the patient, the short dry cough, &c. are in accordance with this view.

When severe pain has been experienced in the epigastric region and towards the back, adhesions have been found between the diaphragmatic and pulmonary pleuræ; but pain is often felt when on examination after death no such adhesions are discovered to enable us to account for it. During the last months of consumption, pain of one or both sides often increases greatly the patient's sufferings.

The pain of the chest which attends catarrh is essentially different in its character; it is referred generally to the centre of the chest, between the sternum and the spine, is felt chiefly during cough, and described as a sense of soreness rather than of pain.

THE PULSE.—The state of the pulse deserves a distinct notice, as much importance has been attached to it. It varies very remarkably, being modified in individual cases by certain physiological and pathological conditions, which may have no direct connexion with the tuberculous disease. Generally speaking, the pulse of the phthisical patient is frequent, especially after the morbid condition of the lungs is fairly established; and in doubtful or obscure cases a frequent pulse would add strongly to our suspicions of the existence of tubercles in the lungs.

But, before we form any judgment as to the frequency of the pulse, its natural state should, if possible, be ascertained in every case. Eighty pulsations in the minute, which may be the natural number in one patient, is a frequent pulse in another whose natural pulse is sixty or sixty-five. In my opinion, the average natural frequency of the pulse in adults is generally estimated too high by authors. Many persons of the tuberculous constitution have habitually a slow, languid circulation, which in some cases continues after there is clear evidence of tuberculous disease of the lungs.

The degree of strength of the pulse also deserves attention; according to my observation it is very generally feeble in persons predisposed to consumption.

Without desiring, therefore, to fix the value of the state of the pulse as a sign of incipient consumption, it always deserves the attention of the physician. A frequent pulse, even taken as an isolated symptom, should excite suspicion; and when accompanied with other symptoms indicative of tuberculous disease, it strongly favours the presumption that mischief has already commenced. On the other hand, a natural state of the pulse may be considered an encouraging circumstance, inasmuch as it is usually associated with a condition of the system favourable to the patient's recovery; while it affords some evidence that the lungs are not extensively tuberculous, and that there is neither much pulmonary nor gastric irritation.

HECTIC FEVER. — The fever which attends phthisis is usually slow and insidious on its first onset, and is, for some time, so slight as often to escape observation. It varies greatly in degree in different cases throughout the whole course of the disease, and is more modified by collateral and accidental affections than perhaps any other symptom. The accidental occurrences to which I allude, are inflammation of the respiratory organs, and gastric and intestinal irritation, which appear to have almost more influence in exciting and modifying the fever than the primary tuberculous disease, which frequently exists for a long period without being attended by an appreciable degree of fever.

The first febrile symptom remarked by the patient is a sensation of chilliness in the evenings. The intensity of this sensation increases with its recur-

rence, amounting often to a slight shivering; it is
then usually succeeded by heat of skin during the
night, the heat being particularly felt in the hands
and feet, which in tuberculous patients are for the
most part habitually cold. After a time morning perspirations succeed the febrile state. As the disease
advances, the paroxysms of fever become stronger,
especially the hot stage, and the heat is more
generally diffused over the surface.

PERSPIRATION.—Although this very prominent
symptom forms a part of the febrile paroxysm, it
is generally so disproportionate to the cold and hot
stages by which it is preceded, and exercises so
great an influence on the feelings of the patient
and the course of the disease, as to merit distinct
consideration.

The fever has generally continued a considerable
time, and the disease is far advanced, before perspiration becomes copious;—in some cases it is entirely
absent. Louis found it wanting in one-tenth of his
cases, and I have met with a few instances of the
same kind. According to the observation of this
physician, the stage of the disease at which the very
copious perspirations occurred, corresponded generally with that at which the diarrhœa made its
appearance. These two affections have commonly
been considered supplementary of each other, the
one diminishing as the other increased. This may
occasionally be the case; but it is not the common

rule, as both in general proceed apparently unin-
fluenced by each other. Louis paid particular
attention to the reputed reciprocal influence of
these two symptoms in other diseases as well as in
phthisis; but he could never find that any such
reciprocal influence existed.

The perspiration occurs chiefly in the mornings,
more especially if the patient happens to fall asleep
after having once awoke. As the disease advances,
it recurs whenever the patient sleeps. During
the early stages, it is generally confined to the
head and chest, but by degrees extends over the
whole surface. I have observed it limited to the
anterior surface of the body, and in many cases to
the head, neck, and chest. The copious perspiration of the consumptive patient presents, as Louis
observes, a remarkable instance of extensive and
long-continued derangement of the function of the
skin, without any appreciable alteration of structure;
and it is very probable that if we could submit the
fluid to examination, it would present characters very
different from those of healthy perspiration. Although
generally occurring in an advanced stage of phthisis,
perspiration occasionally attends its very early
periods; but it is seldom copious at the commencement, and the patient, unless questioned on the
subject, takes little notice of it. After having continued for some time, it not unfrequently ceases
and again recurs, without our being able to account

for such irregularity. In feeble young persons, the copious morning perspiration is one of the most remarkable symptoms, and may be considered an unfavourable omen, as indicating that the disease will run its course rapidly.

The importance of the perspiration as a diagnostic sign is not considerable, because other symptoms of a more marked character usually precede and accompany it; but at the same time it is never to be neglected or passed over with indifference in doubtful cases. I have in a few instances found perspiration, a frequent pulse, and emaciation the only symptoms of pulmonary disease. Whenever we meet with this symptom in a tuberculous constitution, it ought to excite our suspicions and lead us to examine the state of the chest with attention.

THIRST.—This is not a remarkable symptom. It rarely exists to a very great degree, although I have seldom seen it absent. Louis found it wanting in one-fourth of his cases; and where it occurred, it appeared to be more dependent on the fever than on the condition of the digestive organs.

DIARRHŒA.—This is so common an attendant on consumption, as to have been with justice considered one of the most important of its symptoms, exerting apparently a greater influence over its progress than any other; the emaciation, the debility, and consequently the rapidity of the disease being generally proportionate to the severity of the diarrhœa. In all Louis' cases, the wasting and loss of strength corresponded with the number and frequency of the evacuations. This fact suggests a wholesome and not unnecessary caution on the employment of active purgatives even in the early stages of consumption, and of mild aperients in large doses as the disease advances; since they reduce the patient's strength, and may bring on diarrhœa before it would otherwise have occurred. I have seen a table-spoonful of castor-oil throw a phthisical patient into an alarming state of debility.

In persons who have been long constipated, and whose bowels it has been extremely difficult to regulate so as to procure healthy biliary secretions, it is often remarkable how regular their action becomes, and how natural the evacuations are, after phthisis has made some progress.

Diarrhœa seldom occurs until the disease is far advanced, and in a small proportion of cases a few days only before death; sometimes it is entirely wanting. In one-eighth of his cases, Louis found diarrhœa commence with the disease and continue till death; in the majority it occurred in the latter stages; in others during the last days of life only; and in four among one hundred and twelve cases, it never appeared. It often proves one of the most distressing symptoms, being attended, after some time, with severe pains before, and by a deadly sensation of sinking immediately after, each evacuation. The evacuations are generally of a yellow bilious colour.

Although the diarrhœa has no influence in abating the perspiration, it occasionally has an evident effect on the cough and expectoration, diminishing the frequency of the former and the quantity of the latter.

As a diagnostic symptom, diarrhœa is not of much importance, because long before it occurs the nature of the disease is sufficiently evident.

EMACIATION.—When the progress of the disease is not fatally interrupted by some accidental occurrence, few persons die of consumption without being reduced to a great degree of emaciation. In some cases the wasting is the first circumstance which attracts the attention of the patient's friends; in others the disease makes considerable progress before the patient becomes visibly thinner; examples of which I have found most frequently in young females. The cases in which the emaciation becomes extensive before any marked symptom of pulmonary disease occurs, are most common in persons pretty far advanced in life, and in whom the disease has been induced by irregular or unhealthy modes of living, by which the various functions employed in nutrition and assimilation have been impaired. In general, the emaciation begins early, and arises probably in part from the process of assimilation being impeded by the disease of the lungs. The diarrhœa being once established, the process of wasting advances more rapidly, affecting the whole of the soft parts ; and frequently before death there remains little more than the integuments and the bony skeleton.

As a symptom of tuberculous disease, emaciation merits especial attention in obscure cases. In persons about the middle period of life, from forty to fifty, I have found it one of the earliest symptoms of consumption, even when there was no frequency of pulse, no cough, no marked dyspnœa, nor any other symptom to draw attention to the state of the lungs. The derangement of the digestive organs generally present in such cases, is regarded as the principal cause of emaciation ; yet, in spite of all that is done to maintain them in a healthy state and to supply abundant nourishment, it continues to make progress ; and it is not till this state of things has continued for some time that the patient has evening chills, that the pulse becomes frequent, and occasional night perspirations occur.

Emaciation should never be disregarded when there is no evident cause for it. If it is accompanied by quick pulse and loss of strength, and especially if there is any oppression or frequency of breathing, I agree with Louis in believing that tuberculous disease of the lungs rarely fails to prove its cause.

ŒDEMA.—This symptom occurs in general only

towards the termination of phthisis, although it
occasionally appears in a slight degree at an early
period. This is frequently the case in young delicate females, who, in their best health, are often
subject to a degree of œdema, especially in warm
weather.

There is nothing in the œdema of phthisis different from what is remarked in other chronic
diseases, except that it is an invariable attendant ;
at least I have never found it wanting in the last
stage. Although it is chiefly confined to the lower
extremities, and seldom extends higher than the
legs, it is sometimes observed in the arms ; and the
face is frequently œdematous in the mornings
during the last weeks of the disease. Œdema of
the lungs, also, occasionally supervenes in the last
stages, and in other cases an œdematous state of the
glottis. As a diagnostic symptom, œdema is of
little importance, because for the most part the
nature of the disease is well marked long before
its occurrence. In general, however, it is a sure
prognostic that the disease is approaching its termination.

APHTHÆ.—An aphthous state of the mouth is
commonly the last in the long catalogue of maladies which affect the consumptive patient. It occurs generally a week or two before death, and,
like the other symptoms, varies greatly in degree,
being sometimes productive of little inconvenience,

and at others attended with so much irritation and tenderness of the mouth and throat as to prove a source of considerable suffering. The approach of aphthæ is generally marked by a red shining appearance of the tongue, mouth, and fauces, though occasionally they appear with very little redness of the mucous membrane.

There are other symptoms which occasionally attend the progress of consumption, and which may be noticed in this place. An incurvated state of the nails, with a rounded appearance of the last joint of the fingers, is very often observed, and is generally regarded as a diagnostic sign of some importance. The falling-off of the hair is also a common occurrence. The condition of the nervous system undergoes a considerable change : — the patient' becomes nervous, both mentally and physically, even in the early period of the disease : he is timid, and apprehensive of the least circumstance which can increase his complaint : his hand shakes, and he often becomes peevish and irritable. These nervous affections generally keep pace with the increasing debility. The intellect, however, for the most part remains clear till within a few days of death, when slight delirium, as already mentioned, occasionally supervenes.

SECT. II.—PHYSICAL SIGNS.

In the very early stage of tuberculous disease of the lungs we can scarcely expect to derive much positive information from the physical signs, because the tuberculous matter which is present in these organs may not be sufficient to modify in a sensible degree the physical phenomena accompanying the action of respiration. It is quite clear that the vesicular structure of a portion of the lungs must be affected to a degree capable of altering the sounds which accompany healthy respiration, before they can be cognizable to our senses. Persons possessed of a delicate sense of hearing, and whose ear has been well practised in the varying characters of the respiratory sounds, may detect a difference much earlier than is generally supposed; but this degree of nicety cannot be expected from the ordinary auscultator. Those, however, who have endeavoured to ridicule the stethoscope because it does not enable us to detect tuberculous disease at the early period we are now contemplating, could have possessed neither a right conception of the principles upon which the physical signs of pulmonary disease depend, nor a correct knowledge of the anatomy of incipient tubercles. They might as justly deny the powers and utility of the telescope because it does not enable us to discover all the minute phenomena of the starry heavens. Those, also, who venture to affirm that auscultation is useless until the disease is rendered evident by the common symptoms, are equally in error. It is true that auscultation *alone* is often insufficient to detect the disease at a very early period; yet, even at this time, the information which it affords is very valuable, both in a negative and positive point of view. When it does not give us positive assurance of tuberculous disease, it generally enables us to say that, if present, it exists in a very limited extent. In doubtful cases, therefore, we should never fail to examine the sounds of respiration and the degree of resonance of the upper parts of the chest. If both are natural, and alike on both sides, we may feel tolerably certain that tuberculous disease does not exist, or is very limited; if, on the contrary, they differ, we may ascertain the presence of disease which the ordinary symptoms would scarcely lead us to suspect: in a few cases I have even found pectoriloquy, when neither the appearance of the patient nor the symptoms led me to anticipate it. I therefore hold it wise to avail ourselves of auscultation in all cases. It will often assist us powerfully in our diagnosis, and can never lead into error when its results are taken in conjunction with our other means of diagnosis.

The following method of proceeding, while it will be the least formidable to the patient, will enable us most readily to discover the presence and site of tuberculous disease.

RESPIRATORY MOVEMENTS.—In examining the chest, it is of importance to do so with as little parade as may be; otherwise, if the patient is nervous, the respiratory movements may be so imperfectly performed that we shall be unable to obtain any satisfactory information from them. It will also be advantageous to adopt a certain order in our examinations. We should first observe carefully the state of ordinary respiration, and afterwards, by placing the patient fairly before us, mark accurately if the chest is raised equally on both sides during a full inspiration. A difference in this respect will frequently lead us to the seat of the most extensive disease, which exists for the most part on that side which is least raised.

PERCUSSION.—This may next be resorted to, below the clavicles and over the inner extremity of these bones, in order to compare the sound of the chest with that of a healthy one (with which we suppose the auscultator to be acquainted); and also the sound of one side with the other. In most cases mediate is preferable to direct percussion; it is far more agreeable to the patient, and if carefully performed affords equally correct information. Various substances have been used as pleximeters :

that which appears best suited for the purpose is a
piece of flat caoutchouc ; but perhaps the best, and
the only one I employ, is the finger; it conveys
the sound with perfect clearness, and at the same
time removes any fear of pain on the part of
the patient. To perform percussion well, either
the back or fore-part of the finger may be ' pressed
firmly on the chest ; it should then be struck smart-
ly but lightly with the points of two or three fingers
of the other hand ; to effect this, very little force is
required ; in children or young spare persons, the
point of a single finger is sufficient. This simple
operation will, with few exceptions, afford us all
the information to be derived from percussion.   It is
not, however, by any means so easily done as is commonly believed, and consequently it is often imperfectly performed.   The points particularly requiring
attention are, to keep the finger in close contact
with the chest, to strike it at the same angle
wherever applied, and to do this so as to elicit the
resonance, not merely of the parietes, but of the
contents of the chest.   In judging of the sonoriety
of the chest, the thinness of the parietes must be
taken into account; otherwise in the case of children
and very thin persons we may be led into error.

AUSCULTATION.—Having ascertained the resonance of the chest, we next proceed to examine
the respiratory murmur, either with the unaided
ear, or through the medium of the stethoscope.

Although the ear alone is sufficient to examine most
parts of the chest, there are some situations in
which the stethoscope is necessary; such as immediately below and above the clavicles in some
persons, and the axillæ in all. There are other
objections to the application of the ear—some referable to the patient, others to the auscultator,
which are sufficiently obvious. On the back and
sides, however, where the form of the chest admits
of it, the ear is generally preferable; but, assuredly, he who can use the ear and the stethoscope
with equal facility and effect, possesses advantages which are denied to the auscultator who can
use one of them only; and when we hear it stated
that the ear answers all the purposes of the stethoscope, we may safely conclude that the advocates
of that opinion are not very minute in their investigations.

VALUE OF THE PHYSICAL SIGNS.—It is obvious
that tuberculous disease must occupy a considerable portion of the lungs to be capable of in-
fluencing to a perceptible degree the motions of
the chest; simple *inspection* is not, therefore, of
great value in the very early stage, but it is often
useful, and not unfrequently points out the chief
seat of the disease when more advanced.

Percussion, likewise, is of little value at this
period, as tuberculous disease may exist even to
a considerable extent, if the surrounding pulmo-

nary tissue is healthy, without being detected by
it; the sound elicited may even be clearer than
that over a more healthy portion of the lung, which
is the case when the pulmonary vesicles are dilated,
as they often are, amid groups of small tubercles.
Hence, by trusting to percussion alone, we might
be led to consider the diseased as the sound part
of the lung; and the greater the extent of the
emphysematous portion, the more liable are we to
fall into this error. In such cases, by percussing
carefully, we shall sometimes find a small spot,
the dull sound of which contrasts remarkably with
that of the surrounding emphysematous parts.

When the disease is farther advanced, and the
tubercles have coalesced so as to form a solid mass,
or when the pulmonary tissue immediately surrounding them is rendered impermeable to the air by the
effects of inflammation, a dull sound is perceptible,
which, if it exists in the upper part of the chest
only, may be considered as indicating very generally
the presence of tubercles.

Auscultation affords more valuable and precise
information than that derived from the movements
or resonance of the thorax; but in order to obtain
the full advantage of it, we must employ it
with circumspection, as various circumstances may
make it deceptive. A morbid condition of the
mucous membrane from frequent attacks of catarrh,
or what has been termed by Laennec " the dry

catarrh," or an emphysematous state of the lung, may render the respiratory murmur obscure, and lead to the belief that the lung is consolidated. Percussion, however, will enable us to avoid both errors : in the first case it elicits the natural sound, in the latter a particularly clear, or even tympanitic sound. Emphysema is a more frequent source of error than is usually imagined. Portions of the lung are very frequently emphysematous, both in phthisical and other patients, particularly in those subject to chronic coughs, or whose breathing is habitually laborious ; and without keeping this in view, we may be led into error in forming our diagnosis. In these cases, with the obscure respiratory murmur, or in its absence we have the clear sound on percussion, and often a more elevated or rounded form of the chest over the emphysematous portion of lung ; and if the emphysema exists more on one side than on the other, this form of the chest is more evident, particularly in phthisical subjects, in whom the chest usually falls in under the clavicles. A little attention to these circumstances will soon enable the young auscultator to discriminate them.

¹ When the presence of tubercles is suspected, we should examine with the greatest care the clavicular and supra-scapular regions. If the respiration be soft, and free from any rhonchus in these parts, ¿ if it be the same on both sides, and if the

resonance of the voice be also equal, we have strong evidence that there is no tuberculous disease in that part of the lungs where it is most frequently found, or, if it does exist, that it is to a very small extent only.

If the tubercles are diffused generally through the summit of one lung, the resonance of the voice becomes rather stronger, and the respiratory murmur is simply rendered somewhat bronchial and less soft. If, on the other hand, they are considerable in number and confined to a portion of the upper lobe, the natural respiratory murmur is in a great degree lost, the respiration being almost entirely bronchial. In such cases the resonance of the voice also is much louder over the diseased than over the sound portion of lung, amounting often to what is termed bronchophony. As tubercles are almost constantly present to a greater extent on one side of the chest than on the other, the difference of the signs on the two sides will, in obscure cases, greatly assist us in our diagnosis.

Although I have pointed out the upper part as that which requires to be most minutely examined, the examination should be extended over the whole chest; as the symptoms may be produced by chronic pleurisy or chronic pneumonia, the signs of which must be looked for in the condition of the lower part. The upper lobes, although most frequently, are not always the primary seat of tubercles; hence, in obscure cases, we should not venture to form a diagnosis until we ascertain the state of the respiration over the whole chest. In doing this we should not expose the chest; it may be covered with a cotton or flannel dress, which it will be necessary, in some cases only, to remove from the clavicular regions, where the examination should always be made with the greatest care.

I do not hesitate to express my conviction that by adopting a rigid examination on being first consulted, the greater number of cases of tuberculous phthisis would be discovered at a much earlier period of their course,—often, I am persuaded, many months, nay occasionally years, before they now are, from the careless manner in which this class of patients is too commonly examined. Until we adopt a more minute and methodical system of inquiry into the history of the case, and, in addition to the usual symptoms of pulmonary disease, avail ourselves of the light afforded by auscultation, in the most extended sense of that term, tuberculous disease of the lungs can scarcely be detected at such an early period as will give reason to hope that its further progress may be checked. In the present superficial mode of inquiry it is too often far advanced when the patient is said to be merely threatened with it; and tracheal or bronchial irritation are the terms employed to account for symptoms which a closer investigation would trace to a deeper source. We must not be satisfied with a few rough and slovenly thumps on the upper part of the chest, or even with the use of the ear or stethoscope for a few moments, applied as if we were afraid rather than desirous of ascertaining the real condition of the lungs. Such superficial examination, if it deserves the name, is worse than useless : with the semblance of doing something, it really effects nothing, unless it be to deceive the patient and his friends, and bring this method of diagnosis into unmerited disrepute. The examination must be conducted in a very different manner if we expect to derive useful information from it. Nature will not be thus interrogated ; her operations must be closely observed and studied with attention, before we can hope rightly to interpret them.

The physical signs which characterise the different stages of tuberculous consumption have been already detailed when describing the progress of the disease.*

---

* For a detailed account of the *Physical Signs*, I beg to refer the young auscultator to Dr. Williams' work on the *Pathology and Diagnosis of Diseases of the Chest*. Third edition. *London*, 1835.

CHAPTER IV.

As the nature of tubercles was unknown in the early ages of medical science, it is not surprising that the morbid anatomy of pulmonary consumption should have remained so long obscure, and so little understood. Medical writers previously to the seventeenth century adopted the theories of Hippocrates and Galen; regarding tubercles as putrefied phlegm, and ulceration of the lungs as produced by the descent of humours from the head, and the changes of blood effused into the lungs. Sylvius de la Boe, whose works were published in 1679, was the first who gave a good account of tubercles, pointing them out as a cause of phthisis, and showing their connexion with scrofula. He attributed their origin to the scrofulous degeneration of certain invisible glands in the lungs, similar to those in the neck and mesentery.* His opinions were adopted and

* Opera Medica, p. 692.

illustrated by several of his successors, particularly
by Morton and Wepfer, and have been revived in
our own day by Broussais. Nothing more was
known concerning tubercles till the comprehensive
and satisfactory essay of Desault, of Bordeaux,
was published in 1733.* This author, having applied himself during a period of thirty-six years
to the investigation of phthisis, acquired an extensive knowledge of the morbid anatomy of the disease. He maintained that the formation of tubercles
in the lungs was the sole cause of phthisis, and
pointed out many of the facts regarding their development, the discovery of which has been attributed to more recent authors. In the middle of
the last century Russel, Tralles, Gilchrist, and
Mudge, adopted, more or less, the views of Desault ; while their contemporaries neglected or
forgot his discoveries. With these exceptions, the
knowledge of tubercles seems to have retrograded
rather than advanced, till the labours of our indefatigable and accurate countryman Stark, in whose
early death Medicine sustained a serious loss. By
his own careful and minute researches, he acquired
a surprising knowledge of the morbid anatomy of
tuberculous consumption ; and, judging from what
he effected during his short career, there can be
little doubt, had he lived, that he would have anti

* Dissertations de Médecine.

cipated our continental neighbours, even in their minute pathological discoveries.*

Since Stark's time the works of Baillie, and still more those of Bayle, Laennec, Louis, Andral, and Carswell, have rendered our knowledge of the morbid anatomy of tubercles more complete than that of any other morbid product. Various opinions, however, are still entertained respecting their production, their primary site, and the mode in which the various changes they undergo are effected. On these subjects I shall derive great assistance from the labours of Dr. Carswell, whose pathological researches I consider of the greatest importance, as illustrative of tuberculous disease generally.†

SECT. I. THE SEAT, CONSISTENCE, FORM, AND CHEMICAL COMPOSITION OF TUBERCULOUS MATTER.

Minute and careful anatomical researches, often repeated, have led Dr. Carswell to the conclusion

---

* *Stark*, Clinical and Anatomical Observations and Experiments.

† See his *Illustrations of the Elementary Forms of Disease,* Fasc. TUBERCLE; and his article on the same subject in the *Cyclopædia of Practical Medicine,* which together contain a full pathological history of tubercle.

that the surfaces of the mucous and serous tissues, and the blood, form the exclusive *seat* of tuberculous matter. In no instance has he found this morbid product deposited in the molecular structure of organs. The free surface of mucous membranes forms the chief seat of tuberculous deposits. "There, as into the great emunctory of the system, it appears to be separated from the blood and becomes visible to us under a variety of forms." " In whatever organ the formation of tuberculous matter takes place, the mucous system, if constituting a part of that organ, is in general either the exclusive seat of this morbid product, or is far more extensively affected with it than any of the other systems or tissues of the same organ."* But in those organs in which the mucous tissue is minutely distributed, as in the lungs, it is often difficult to demonstrate the presence of tuberculous matter in this system, and the more rapid its deposition the greater is the difficulty; and this is still farther increased when such deposit is complicated with inflammation.

The free surfaces of serous membranes and the cellular tissue in general form the frequent seat of tubercle.

" As a morbid constituent of the blood," Dr. Carswell observes, " we can take no cognizance of the

---

* Dr. Carswell, op. citat. art. TUBERCLE.

existence of tubercles, otherwise than through the medium of the secretions, or until that fluid has ceased to circulate; then the tuberculous matter is seen to separate from the serum, fibrin, and colouring matter, and is distinguished from them by its peculiar physical characters." In this state it is met with in the cells of the spleen.

The *consistence* of tuberculous matter varies from that of a fluid. to the firmness of cheese ; the degree of consistence depending chiefly on the resistance offered to its accumulation and the absorption of its more fluid parts.

The *form* of tuberculous matter Dr. Carswell considers as entirely dependent on the structure of the organ in which it is deposited. Its granular appearance in the lungs is owing to its accumulation in a small number of contiguous air-cells ; and the lobular arrangement, which it sometimes presents in the same organ, is produced by its being deposited in the air-cells of a number of lobules, the intervening pulmonary tissue being unaffected. When the tuberculous matter is disseminated throughout a considerable extent of lung, it has no definite form.

Whatever may be the site, consistence, or form of tuberculous matter, it is to be regarded as a morbid inorganizable product, and consequently insusceptible of any change that is not effected by the living tissue in which it is deposited.

Animal chemistry has not done much to illustrate the nature of tuberculous deposits, and a rich field of inquiry on this subject is still open to the experimental chemist. It would be very desirable to have the blood and other fluids of tuberculous subjects analyzed, as well as tuberculous deposits in man at different ages, and also in the lower animals.

The chemical composition of tuberculous matter varies according to the different periods at which it is examined, also in different animals, and probably in different organs. In man it is chiefly composed of albumen with varying proportions of gelatine and fibrine.*

SECT. II.—MORBID ANATOMY OF PULMONARY TUBERCLE.

Tuberculous matter is deposited in the lungs in three distinct forms,—grey semi-transparent gra-

---

* Coloured representations of the varieties of form assumed by tuberculous matter in different organs, are given in the first fasciculus of the *Illustrations of the Elementary Forms of Disease*, now publishing by Dr. Carswell; a work which, whether we regard its beauty and fidelity of execution, or its importance and utility in a pathological point of view, far surpasses any thing of the kind that has been produced in this or any other country.

nulations,—caseous or crude tubercle,—and tuberculous infiltration.

Granulations.—Grey semi-transparent granulations are scarcely ever absent in any form or stage
of consumption. Their consistence approaches
that of cartilage ; they are generally grey, though
sometimes colourless, and vary in size from that of a
mustard-seed to that of a pea, being sometimes distinct, sometimes united in small grape-like clusters,
and more rarely agglomerated in larger masses.
They are most commonly found in considerable
numbers, often occupying a great part of the tissue
around large excavations and the bands which tra-
verse them. The period required for their development is very variable. In acute phthisis, Louis
says they may reach the size of a pea in three of
four weeks. When subjects already labouring
under consumption, or who are in a state of
tuberculous cachexia, are exposed to violent irri-
tations of the lungs, these granulations are deposited so rapidly and in such numbers throughout
the lungs, as to give rise to the most alarming
dyspnœa. In other cases they may remain small for
a considerable period; thus, in several individuals
who had cough and frequent attacks of hemoptysis
for many years, granulations, about the size of
peas, were the only lesion found by Louis after
death.

The granulations, after a time, begin to lose

their transparency and consistence, and become
white, opaque, and friable; in which state they
receive the name of crude tubercles. The period at
which these changes take place varies indefinitely;
from the observations of Papavoine,* Tornelle,†
&c., it would appear that the change is more
rapid in children than in adults : Louis met with
five adults in whom the granulations were unal-
tered. .Laennec and Louis suppose that the change
begins invariably at the centre of the granulations;
but Andral and Carswell maintain that it may
begin at the centre or at any point of the circumference indifferently.

Grey granulations were first observed and described by Bayle, who thought they were a morbid
product, *sui generis.* He described them as constituting a species of consumption, sometimes
entirely simple, but most commonly complicated
with the tuberculous. He supposed that in time
they produce ulceration, and that the caverns to
which they give rise are distinguished from those
which follow tubercles by being lined with false
membrane. Laennec, on the other hand, maintained that they are necessarily the first form under
which tubercle presents itself; and Louis and some
other pathologists have adopted Laennec's views.
But Dr. Carswell shows that the grey semi-trans-

---

* Journ. des Progrès.   † Journ. Hebdomadaire.

parent substance does not necessarily precede the formation of opaque tuberculous matter; that the latter is found in several organs in which granulations are never observed; and that the granular form chiefly depends on the structure of the air-cells in which it is deposited.

Crude tubercle.—This term is applied to certain tumours of a rounded form, varying in size from that of a pin's head to that of a small walnut. They have a yellowish white colour and a soft cheesy consistence. They are, as has been stated, generally the result of changes which have taken place in the matter deposited under the form of grey granulations: but these two forms almost always co-exist, Louis having met with only two cases of crude tubercle without granulations, and five of granulations without tubercles.

Tuberculous infiltration.—The third form in which tuberculous matter presents itself in the lungs is that of infiltration into the cellular tissue of the organ. Baillie, who first noticed this state, gives the following accurate account of it:—" In cutting into the lungs, a considerable portion of their structure sometimes appears to be changed into a whitish soft matter, somewhat intermediate between a solid and a fluid, like a scrofulous gland just beginning to suppurate. This appearance is, I believe, produced by scrofulous matter being deposited in the cellular substance of a certain portion of the lungs, and advancing towards suppuration. It seems to be the same matter with that of tubercle, but only diffused uniformly over a considerable portion of the lungs, while the tubercle is circumscribed."* This has since been described by French authors under the name of ' infiltration.'

Another deposit of a peculiar kind, never found in other diseases, is the yellow jelly-like matter, the ' infiltration tuberculeuse gélatiniforme' of Laennec, who believes that it is only a more liquid state of the tuberculous matter poured into the parenchyma of the lungs;—an opinion which I am inclined to adopt, from having seen large quantities of a similar matter, containing small isolated flakes of crude tubercles, deposited around a scrofulous joint.

The nature, extent, and relation of the different forms of tuberculous matter, and the changes which they undergo in the lungs, vary greatly in different cases. In general, tuberculous matter first makes its appearance in the lungs in the form of grey semi-transparent granulations, gradually takes on the characters of crude tubercle, and ultimately becomes softened. During the process of softening and ulceration, tuberculous matter continues to be deposited in other portions of the lung, the progress being generally from above downwards; so that we

* Morbid Anatomy.

often find excavations at the summit, crude or
softened tubercles below these, and granulations,
with no trace of opaque matter, in the lowest part.
At a late period of the disease the substance of
the lung is often so filled with tuberculous matter
as to leave but few traces of its original structure,
the whole constituting a mass of dull, opaque,
grey, or white tubercular infiltration, excavated to
a greater or less extent.

The upper and back part of the lungs is the
most common seat of tubercle, and the left side
is more frequently affected than the right,—an
observation first made by Stark, and corrobo-
rated by Carmichael Smyth from an examination
of the cases recorded by Bonetus and Morgagni,
and more recently by Louis from his own experience. The last author found tubercles exclusively
confined to the right side in two cases only, and
in five to the left: of thirty-eight, in which the
upper lobe was totally occupied by large excavations and tubercles, so as to be impermeable to
air, he met with twenty-eight in the left and ten
only in the right lung; and in eight of perforation of the pleura, he found seven on the left and
one only on the right side. When to these observations we add the result of Reynaud's experience,
who, of forty cases of pneumothorax, found twenty-
seven on the left side, and thirteen only on the
right, I consider that there is sufficient evidence

to confirm the conclusion that the left lung is most frequently affected.* This is the reverse of the relative frequency of pneumonia, on the two sides, at all ages. M. Lombard found that, of eight hundred and sixty-eight cases of pneumonia, four hundred and thirteen were affected on the right side only, two hundred and sixty on the left, and one hundred and ninety-five on both sides. By the above comparison it appears that pneumonia on the right side is, to that on the left, in point of frequency, as three to two.†

Softening of tubercle. — By those, who, with Laennec, regard tubercle as organizable, the process of softening has been considered a consequence of the death of this substance ; and by others, who do not take this view of the subject, it has been stated to begin always at the centre and to proceed towards the circumference. But Dr. Carswell has shown that the softer appearance of the centre of the tubercle has no connexion with the process of softening. It depends on the tuberculous matter being deposited upon the internal surface only of the air-vesicles or bronchi, the central portion being occupied by mucus or other secreted fluids. When the air-cells or minute bronchi, thus partially filled with tuberculous matter, are divided,

* Journ Hebdomadaire, vol. vii. p. 61.
† Archives Gén. de Méd. t. xxv. p. 60.

they represent tubercles with softening in the
central point; when, on the other hand, they
are completely filled, no such appearance is presented. " Softening," Dr. Carswell further observes, " begins most frequently at the circumference of firm tuberculous matter, or where its
presence, as a foreign body, is most felt by the
surrounding tissues. In the lungs and cellular
structure of other parts it is often seen making its
appearance in several points of an agglomerated
mass of tubercle, which has included within it
portions of the tissue in which it was deposited ;
whereas, in the brain, the substance of which
has, from the commencement, been separated and
pushed outwards by the tuberculous matter, the
softening process begins, and is always most marked
on the circumference." The softening of tuberculous matter is therefore to be regarded merely as
a consequence of the changes excited in the living
tissues in which this matter is deposited. The
parts in immediate contact with the tubercle pour
out serosity and take on the ulcerative action, by
which the tuberculous matter is sooner or later
softened and expectorated, leaving in its place a
cavity, which, by the successive softening and
expectoration of contiguous tuberculous masses,
becomes gradually increased in size. Before these
changes take place, tubercle appears to produce
little disturbance in the general economy, and may

exist for some time in several organs attended by symptoms so slight as scarcely to indicate its presence.

State of the lung around tubercles.—Dr. Carswell has remarked it as an important fact that the mucous and serous tissues in contact with tuberculous matter are often found in a healthy condition. While this continues, tubercles may remain for an indefinite length of time in their original state; or the softer part of the tubercle may be absorbed, leaving the more solid calcareous portion only in its site; a termination which occurs more commonly, I believe, than is generally supposed.

Much more frequently the surrounding pulmonary tissue is found in a morbid state.

The changes induced by the presence of tubercles are, serous and sanguineous congestion, inflammation, induration, or softening, ulceration, mortification, atrophy, and the formation of accidental tissues of a fibrous or cartilaginous nature.

Serous congestion, according to Dr. Carswell's observation, occurs most frequently in those cases in which the tuberculous matter is rapidly deposited in the lungs to a considerable extent, as occurs in the acute febrile form of phthisis already described. The serous infiltration of the pulmonary tissue around the tubercular granulations increases greatly the dyspnœa by impeding the free admission of air into the lungs.

Sanguineous congestion occurs to a greater or less extent in every case. Dr. Carswell remarks that when the tuberculous matter is situated at the root of the lungs, the large pulmonary veins may be compressed so as to prevent a free return of blood to the heart, and thus produce general pulmonary congestion. In other parts of the lungs, the congestion which arises from the presence of tubercles is only partial. In either case hemoptysis may be the consequence; but it is equally certain that, when considerable, it is very commonly attended with general and active congestion of the lungs, and often occurs before the accumulation of tuberculous matter is sufficiently extensive to produce much obstruction to the circulation through the larger vessels.

When, instead of producing merely impeded circulation and consequent congestion of the lungs, tubercles give rise to irritation and inflammation, we have the usual appearances of inflammation in its various grades.

The views of Dr. Carswell, regarding the seat of tubercle, enable us to explain, in a very satisfactory manner, the mode in which the different tissues are successively affected. The tuberculous matter being, as he describes, deposited in the air-vesicles and minute bronchial tubes, these parts are necessarily first irritated by it; and being constantly distended by the matter accumulating within them, they are gradually enlarged in size, and sooner or later are destroyed by ulcerative absorption. Hence it is that the bronchi are always found enlarged, stopping abruptly, and appearing as it were cut across, at their entrance into a cavern. Unlike the other parts of the lungs, they are never found enveloped and compressed by tubercles, except in those instances of rapid infiltration in which the whole substance of the lung appears to be simultaneously injected.

The cellular tissue, healthy air-vesicles, and bloodvessels are at first only pushed aside, and compressed by the tuberculous deposits, but they are ultimately condensed and rendered impervious to air by the infiltration of tuberculous matter and the common products of inflammation.

The mode in which the bloodvessels are affected by the development of tubercles and the formation of caverns in the lungs, has been so well described by Stark, that we cannot refrain from introducing the whole of his remarks upon it. " The pulmonary arteries and veins," he says, " as they approach the larger vomicæ, are suddenly contracted ; a bloodvessel which, at its beginning, measured half an inch in circumference, sometimes (although it had sent off no considerable branch) could not be cut up further than half an inch. And when outwardly they are of a large size, yet internally they have a very small canal, being almost filled up

by a fibrous substance; and frequently, as they pass
along the sides of vomicæ, they are found quite detached, for about an inch of their course, from the
neighbouring parts. That the bloodvessels are thus
obstructed, and that they have little or no communication with the vomicæ, is rendered still more
evident by blowing into them; by blowing they
are not sensibly distended, nor does the air pass
into the vomicæ, excepting very rarely, and then
only by some imperceptible holes: and after injecting the lungs by the pulmonary artery and vein,
the parts less affected by disease, which before injection were the softest, become the hardest, and,
vice versâ, the most diseased parts, before injection
the hardest, are now the softest.

" Upon cutting into the sounder parts, number-
less ramuli may be seen filled with the wax, but in
the diseased parts there is no such appearance;
and upon tracing, by dissection, the injected vessels,
those which terminate in the sounder parts may be
traced a long way to the smaller ramuli; but those
which lead to tubercles and vomicæ a very short
way, and only to their principal branches. The
wax was very rarely found to have entered the
middling-sized vomicæ, and never the smaller or
larger ones."*

Perforation of the coats of the bloodvessels,

* Op. citat. p. 28.

though never observed by Stark, occasionally takes place ; and according to the size of the opening and the capacity of the affected vessel, the patient may have trifling hemoptysis, or perish in a few seconds from the profuse discharge of blood.

Tuberculous cavities generally contain more or less fluid of various consistence and colour ; sometimes having a resemblance to thick curds ; at others to pus, or simple serum, or a mixture of these, and in some instances blood. Cavities are occasionally found quite empty and lined throughout with a dense membrane. This is intimately united with the mucous membrane of the bronchi at the point where the latter enter, and, according to Louis, frequently consists of two layers,—the first, or internal, being dense, grey, or almost semi-transparent and semi-cartilaginous, about the third or fourth of a line in thickness ; the second very soft, yellow or white, of about the same thickness, but often not continued over the whole surface, as the first is. Their density and even their existence often seem to bear a relation to the age of the cavity. Both these layers were wanting in a fourth of the cases examined by Louis, leaving the pulmonary tissue quite bare.

As the neighbouring caverns increase in size, the intervening parenchyma is gradually destroyed, till they coalesce, and an entire lobe may be thus converted into one large, jagged, irregular cavity, in

which portions of pulmonary tissue are often found,
either hanging loosely or traversing it in various
directions in the shape of bands, and occasionally
perfectly detached. These loosened portions, the
bands, and the walls of the caverns, present little
or no trace of the healthy pulmonary structure.
They are of a reddish or grey colour, and are exceed-
ingly hard, being for the most part composed of
semi-transparent granulations, or crude tubercle and
black pulmonary matter. Portions of the walls
are also occasionally found in a state of mortification.

The extent to which the lungs are affected by the
progress of tuberculous disease varies greatly. In
some cases a few caverns only are found at the
summit of the lungs; in others the portion of
healthy parenchyma which remains is so exceed-
ingly small as to excite surprise that the function
of respiration could have been carried on so as to
support life. Stark calculated that the extent of
lung which remains fit for the admission of air may
be estimated, at a medium, to be about one-fourth
of the whole substance.

CHAPTER V.

THAT pulmonary consumption admits of a cure is no longer a matter of doubt; it has been clearly demonstrated by the researches of Laennec and other modern pathologists. " Pathological anatomy," says Dr. Carswell, " has perhaps never afforded more conclusive evidence in proof of the curability of a disease than it has in that of tubercular phthisis." I subjoin this author's account of the process by which the cure is effected; it comprehends a description of those changes in the condition of the tuberculous matter, contiguous pulmonary tissue, and bronchi, which indicate that a cure of pulmonary tubercle has taken place.

On examining a portion of lung in which a cure of tuberculous disease has been effected, we find that " the tuberculous matter, whether contained in a bronchial tube, the air-cells, or cellular tissue of the lungs, has assumed a dry, putty-looking, chalky, or cretaceous character. If the tuberculous matter is observed in an excavation, the surrounding pulmonary substance is generally dark-coloured and firm; and if the excavation exists in the course of large bronchial tubes, those situated between the excavation and the surface of the lungs are obliterated, whilst those in the opposite direction terminate either in a shut extremity near the excavation, or are continuous with the lining membrane, or with the accidental tissue which incloses the altered tuberculous matter. The existence of this accidental tissue is an important circumstance as regards the cicatrization of tubercular excavations. It is formed by the effusion of coagulable lymph on the internal surface of the excavation, or into the substance of the contiguous pulmonary tissue; it has, in the former situation, so long as a ready exit is afforded to its secretion, the characters of simple mucous tissue; but at a later period, and especially when the latter condition is wanting, it becomes gradually and successively converted into serous, fibrous, fibro-cartilaginous, and cartilaginous tissues. The cartilaginous and the osseous transformations of this accidental tissue are, however, rare, particularly the latter. It much more frequently presents and retains the fibrous character, and possesses the property of contracting so as to diminish the bulk of the excavation, and carry with it the pulmonary tissue with which it is connected. The diminution of bulk which accompanies the removal of the tu-

berculous matter, and the contraction of the accidental tissue, give rise to a puckering of the lung,
which is best seen where the pleura has been forced
to follow the retrocession of the pulmonary tissue
beneath it, and around what is called the cicatrix :
for there sometimes remains only a small globular,
oval, or even linear portion of fibrous or fibro-cartilaginous tissue, where, from the extensive puckering of the lung around it, there must have formerly
existed an excavation of considerable extent.

" When the tuberculous matter is contained
within the bronchi, or a cavity formed by the dila-
tation of the air-cells, it does not appear that any
accidental tissue is formed during the cure. The
matter appears to be gradually removed by expectoration, if the bronchi remain pervious, or by absorption if they have become closed ; and then we
have the same obliteration of the terminal branches
already noticed, and the same puckering of the
surrounding tissues. So complete is the cicatrization of a tuberculous excavation in some cases, that
the fibro-cartilaginous substance by which the site
is generally recognized, has entirely disappeared,
and there remains only a small nucleus of cretaceous
matter not larger than a pin's head. Even this, the
remains of the tuberculous matter, may also have
disappeared ; so that, to a common observer, the
pulmonary tissue appears to be in all respects
healthy. But when more narrowly examined, we

perceive that there is a central point towards which the course of several bloodvessels and bronchi is directed. These bloodvessels and bronchi can be traced terminating in this point, either by dissecting them with care, injecting, or inflating them. There are many circumstances, into the details of which we cannot enter, which prove most satisfactorily that the obliteration of the bloodvessels and bronchi in such cases is the consequence of the entire removal of tuberculous matter, and the cicatrization of the cavity in which it was contained.

" The *extent* of the upper lobe of the lung occupied by cretaceous matter and cicatrices varies considerably. Most frequently the presence of one or both is confined to a circumscribed portion of the summit or back part of the lobe. Sometimes cretaceous matter, and cicatrices in various stages of their progress, occupy the upper half or two-thirds of this lobe, and the bronchial glands may, at the same time, present similar appearances. The upper lobe of one lung, or of both lungs, may present these appearances; or, being present on one side, they may be accompanied with tuberculous deposition and excavations on the other side. Lastly, cretaceous matter, cicatrices, or both, may be accompanied by the presence of tuberculous matter and excavations in the same or neighbouring lobe; thus indicating, when the other circumstances already mentioned are taken into account, the dependence of the former on the previous existence of the latter. There must be few practical patholo-' gists who will not consider these anatomical facts as affording sufficient evidence that tuberculous phthisis is curable. These changes are positive indications of the removal of the material element of the disease, and also of the cure of those lesions of structure to which it gives rise even at an advanced period of its progress. The cure of tuberculous disease in other organs has not been so satisfactorily demonstrated. We have, however, as was before done by Dr. Jenner, and since by Dr. Baron, frequently produced tubercles in the liver of a rabbit, and afterwards ascertained that their complete removal was affected by absorption and excretion. When it was accomplished by the latter process, which is most commonly the case, no trace of the disease remained ; and when effected by absorption, the surface of the liver was found marked by irregular furrows or depressions, apparently produced by atrophy of the organ in the site of the tuberculous matter."*

In recording these proofs of the curability of pulmonary tubercles, I think it right to remark that I do not attach much importance to them, further than that they afford encouragement to persevere in our endeavours to correct the tuberculous diathesis ;

* *Cyclopædia of Practical Medicine,*—TUBERCLE.

seeing that nature can remedy the local disease when it is not very extensive. We must never allow our hopes of such a termination of the disease, nor our endeavours to promote it by local remedies, to divert our attention from the constitutional treatment. Unless we can correct the constitutional disorder in which local tuberculous disease has its origin, such cure is of little avail, as it is usually succeeded by fresh deposits of tubercles to an extent which renders recovery hopeless. It not unfrequently happens that young persons are attacked with symptoms of phthisis, which under proper treatment cease, and years elapse before there is any renewal of the disease. Were advantage taken of the intervening period to correct the tuberculous diathesis, the cure might prove perfect. I have known recoveries from two such attacks, the third proving fatal; the interval between the first and last attack was twelve years. The opinion of Laennec on this subject is so important, that I shall cite his words: " We may indeed say, that the greater number of cases of phthisis are latent at the beginning, since we have seen that nothing is more common than to find numerous miliary tubercles in lungs otherwise quite healthy, and in subjects who had never shown any symptoms of consumption. On the other hand, from considering the great number of phthisical and other subjects in whom

cicatrices are found in the summit of the lungs, I
think it is more than probable that hardly any person is carried off by a first attack of phthisis.
Since I was first led to adopt this opinion on anatomical grounds, it has frequently appeared quite
clear to me, from carefully comparing the history
of my patients with the appearances on dissection,
that the greater number of those first attacks are
mistaken for slight colds, and that others are quite
latent, being unaccompanied with either cough or
expectoration, or indeed with any symptoms sufficient to impress the memory of the patients themselves." I am satisfied, from my own observation,
that Laennec's opinion is correct. Tuberculous
disease of the lungs in early life is, I believe,
frequently cured ; but it very generally recurs,
often at an advanced age, and ultimately proves
fatal. The cases of this kind which I have observed have been most frequently in females.
While proper measures, therefore, are adopted to
abate pulmonary irritation and congestion, our
utmost endeavours should be directed to correct
the constitutional disorder, as the only sure means
of obviating a renewal of tuberculous disease.

CHAPTER VI.

As consumption has its origin in a morbid state
of the constitution, we should naturally expect to
find tuberculous disease occurring in various organs,
in the same individual. This is actually the case;
for although the lungs are generally first and most
extensively affected, many other organs become
tuberculous in the course of the disease : indeed,
there is scarcely a part of the body in which tuber-
çles have not been found.

There are also other morbid lesions, particularly
of the mucous membranes, which complicate, and
are so intimately connected with, consumption, as
apparently to form constituent parts of it: and
it is worthy of remark that some of these secondary affections are occasionally so prominent
as to mask the primary and most important affection, which is only made manifest by examination
after death. In some cases, for example, the
diarrhœa is so severe, and assumes so much the

character of chronic dysentery as for a time to throw into the back-ground the less evident symptoms of pulmonary phthisis: but, on examination after death, although the intestines are found ulcerated and otherwise diseased, the lungs are in general so much more affected, as to leave no doubt that they were the primary seat of disease. Again, disease of the larynx occasionally produces such marked symptoms as to be taken for the principal affection, even when the lungs are extensively tuberculous. I shall notice the most important complications.

SECT. I.—DISEASES OF THE ORGANS OF RESPIRATION.

The mucous membrane of the air-passages is generally diseased, in the course of pulmonary consumption, to a greater or less extent.

Ulceration of the epiglottis.—This generally occurs late in the disease. The ulceration, when slight, gives rise to no symptom by which its existence can be known; but in general the larynx is affected at the same time and in the same manner. The lingual surface of the epiglottis is rarely ulcerated; Louis found it so in one case only; the symptoms were, a painful sensation in the region of the os hyoides, and difficult deglutition, fluids being frequently ejected through the nostrils in the attempt to swallow them. This last symptom is considered characteristic of inflamed epiglottis, although it does not always attend it : I have seen it swollen and intensely red, and yet deglutition was not attended with much pain. In some cases the epiglottis becomes œdematous.

Ulceration of the larynx.—This is a frequent concomitant of tuberculous disease of the lungs. It occurs for the most part only in the advanced stages, but occasionally symptoms indicative of its existence make their appearance before the signs of pulmonary affection are very evident. The symptoms depend upon the site of the ulceration, and generally keep pace with its extension. In some cases they are so prominent and attract the attention of both the physician and patient so forcibly, as to lead to the belief that the larynx is the chief seat of the disease, and that the patient labours under laryngeal phthisis. But, as M. Andral justly remarks, the disease which has been designated by that term is in most cases pulmonary consumption accompanied by a morbid condition of the larnyx, the symptoms of which predominate and mask those of the pulmonary disease, upon which the emaciation, hectic fever, and other important symptoms entirely depend. One of the most constant symptoms of ulcerated larynx is hoarseness, which increases often to complete aphonia. More or less pain commonly exists in the region of the os hyoides, being often severe when the ulcerations are deep. The cough has a peculiar character in this affection ; it is accompanied with a harsh, grating sound, and sometimes resembles a kind of whistling.

Ulcerations of the trachea.—These do not give rise to any particular symptoms, and their existence is in general ascertained only by examination after death. Of the many patients examined by Louis, one only complained of a sensation, of heat and obstruction behind and above the sternum :—a great part of the mucous membrane of the fleshy part of the trachea was destroyed by ulceration. In the other cases examined by this accurate pathologist, no symptom could be attributed to the ulcerations, however numerous ; there was no peculiarity either in the cough or in the character of the expectoration. Louis attributes the absence of symptoms in these cases to the slow progress of the disease. When simple inflammation of the mucous membrane of the trachea exists, there is often a sensation of heat and pain. Ulcerations of the trachea are almost exclusively found in phthisical subjects : they are frequently confined to one side, which, according to Andral's observations, invariably corresponds with the diseased lung, or, if both lungs are diseased, with that which is most affected.

The *Bronchial* membrane is found reddened,
much thickened, and sometimes ulcerated. These
changes are, however, chiefly confined to the tubes
in communication with caverns, and, in M. Louis'
opinion, depend upon the passage of the purulent
matter along them, inasmuch as they are seldom
met with in the neighbourhood of unsoftened tubercles or grey granulations, and occur more frequently and to a greater extent near old caverns than
near those of recent formation. Similar changes
which occur in the larynx, trachea, and epiglottis,
appear to M. Louis to be connected with the
passage of the sputa ; since they chiefly affect the
posterior parts of the trachea and larynx, and the
laryngeal surface of the epiglottis, and, as we have
remarked, are scarcely ever found on the lingual
surfaces of the latter, or in the ventricles of the
larynx.

Ulcerations are much more frequent in the larynx
and trachea than in the larger bronchi. Dr. Carswell informs us that they are very common in
the minute ramifications of the bronchi. The
ulcers are generally accompanied with reddening
and thickening of the surrounding membrane,
although Louis has met with instances in which it
was perfectly colourless. The margins of the ulcers
are even and well-defined, and they are generally
so small and superficial as to be detected only by
close examination. At other times they extend the

whole length of the fleshy portion of the trachea,
or along the back of the larynx and under-surface of
the epiglottis. They seldom penetrate deeper than
the mucous membrane, although in some cases
the muscular and cartilaginous rings of the trachea,
the cordæ vocales, the arytenoid cartilages, and
epiglottis are partially involved ; and in one case
observed by Louis the epiglottis was completely
destroyed. Dr. Carswell remarks that tuberculous
matter is not often found in the larynx, in the trachea,
or its larger divisions ; he has met with it in only a
few instances in the follicles of these parts and in
the sacculi laryngis.

The close connexion of these lesions with phthisis
is established by the fact that Louis found ulceration of the epiglottis and larynx in *one-fifth*, and
ulceration of the trachea in *one-third* of the cases
which he examined ; whereas he found it once only
in one hundred and twenty-two patients who died
of other chronic diseases. The same accurate pathologist discovered that these ulcerations occur more
frequently in men than in women, in the proportion
of two to one.

Affections of the pleura.—The morbid changes
which the pleura undergoes during the progress of
tuberculous disease of the lungs consist in the effusion of coagulable lymph on its surface, and consequent adhesion to the pleura costalis. Such adhesions almost constantly accompany the formation

of tubercles, and their extent corresponds with that of the tuberculous disease. In only one case of one hundred and thirteen examined by Louis, both lungs were free from adhesions; the right was exempt in eight cases, and the left in seven : in twenty-eight they were small and easily broken down, and the caverns were either small or wanting. In the other two-thirds, they were dense and firm, and accompanied with large excavations. In two cases, where the lungs contained but two excavations, the adhesions existed only over the parts corresponding with them.

These facts show, in the clearest and most satisfactory manner, the intimate relation of tubercles and adhesions as cause and effect. From the adhesions being often confined to the spot corresponding with the tuberculous excavations, and from the absence of all appreciable signs of inflammation during their formation, it is probable that the lymph of which they are composed is frequently poured out from the vessels with little or no irritative action. They sometimes present the appearance of semi-cartilaginous crusts, covering the summit of the lungs, and in other instances they are changed into true tuberculous matter. If the ulcerative process goes on in the walls of the caverns till the intervening pulmonary tissue and pleura are destroyed, these new formations constitute the proper walls of the caverns; and if

the process advances, these also may be destroyed,
and the matter point externally.

Perforation of the pleura.—One of the most distressing accidents which occur during the progress
of phthisis, is the perforation of the pleura, and
the consequent escape of air and purulent matter
into its cavity. It is characterised by the sudden-
ness of its occurrence and by the marked symptoms to which it gives rise,—sudden pain in the
side affected, great oppression of breathing, and
extreme anxiety, which are speedily followed by
symptoms of acute pleurisy. This accident resembles the perforation of the intestine, the escape of feculent matter into the cavity of the
peritoneum, and the violent inflammation of that
membrane.

Perforation of the pleura for the most part occurs
in the advanced stage of the disease when the
patient's strength is greatly reduced, and in general
proves speedily fatal. It has caused death in
twenty-four hours ; but when the symptoms are
less acute, the patient has lived for thirty days ;
and Dr. Stokes states a case where the patient sur-
vived five months. A sudden attack of pain, on
one side of a phthisical patient, with much oppression and anxiety, may be considered as indicating
the accident. Louis, however, gives a case (xliv.)
where oppression and anxiety, without pain, marked
its occurrence.

Perforation of the pleura may take place under two circumstances :--a tuberculous cavity, which communicates with the pleura by means of the perforation, may or may not communicate with the trachea. In the former case we have generally an effusion of air and fluid into the cavity of the pleura, connected with which there is present a peculiar symptom called *metallic tinkling*, or a clear fine sound resembling that produced by the falling of a pin on glass, and heard when the patient speaks or coughs. When there is no communication between the tuberculous cavity and the pleura and bronchi, or when there is an effusion of air only or a very small quantity of liquid, it was Laennec's opinion that there could be no metallic tinkling. Dr. Williams, however, has shown the fallacy of this opinion, and that neither communication with the bronchi nor liquid effusion is necessary to the production of the phenomenon :—he considers it to be nothing more than an echo or resonance which any sound or impulse propagated to a cavity of a certain form may produce.*

Of eight cases of perforation which occurred to Louis, seven were on the left side,—a circumstance which he attributes to tuberculous disease being more frequent on that side, and often more advanced than on the right.

---

* Op. citat.

Perforation of the pleura generally takes place over a tuberculous abscess or cavern of considerable extent; yet cases occasionally occur in which a small softened tubercle immediately under the pleura bursts and discharges its contents, and this may be one of a very few contained in the lungs. Andral mentions a case of this kind where the lungs contained only five or six tubercles. In such cases, from the small size of the cavity, little or no effusion of pus or other matter takes place, and, consequently, the perforation is not necessarily followed by pleuritis.

Great accumulation of air in the pleura gives rise to the most distressing dyspnœa, and generally soon proves fatal, from impeded respiration. I lately met with a remarkable example of this kind: tuberculous disease was far advanced in the right side, while the left was but little affected; the patient was suddenly attacked after a fit of coughing with severe dyspnœa: the left side was found tympanitic, the intercostal spaces were distended, and no respiratory murmur could be heard. An opening was made between the intercostal space of the fourth and fifth ribs, from which the air rushed out with great violence, giving considerable relief to the patient. Death, however, took place in twelve hours from the commencement of the attack. On opening the body, the right lung was found everywhere adherent and

full of caverns and tubercles; the left was, for the
most part, free; but in one portion a dense though
not extensive adhesion had been partly torn from
its attachment, thereby causing a rupture of the
pleura over a very small tuberculous cavity, through
which the air had passed freely from the bronchi
into ,the chest, giving rise to all the distressing
symptoms. The history of this case affords a good
example of the manner in which the perforation is
sometimes produced. This patient was seized, a
few days before the accident, with acute pain in the
left side of the chest; the pulse was accelerated,
and other symptoms supervened, indicating an attack
of pleuritis, which, being successfully combated
by antiphlogistic treatment, had entirely ceased two
days before the accession of the dyspnœa. From
the weak state of the patient the existence of effusion could not be ascertained during life, but after
death it was found to have taken place to the
extent of twelve or fifteen ounces : by separating
the pulmonary from the costal pleura, it had produced a partial rupture of the cellular tissue which
formed the adhesion, and which was elongated
between the two pleuræ to nearly an inch, and kept
in a state of tension. In this state of the parts,
the succussion of the cough had torn the pulmonary pleura at the edge of the adhesion, and
thus produced the perforation. For this ingenious
explanation of the manner in which effusion may

break up adhesions, and occasionally give rise to perforation, we are indebted to Dr. Carswell.

Inflammation of the lungs and of the pleura and pericardium, is among the most common inter-current diseases which attend and complicate the last stage of phthisis, and not unfrequently cuts off a patient, in a few days, who might otherwise have lived for weeks, or even months.

SECT. II.—DISEASES OF THE ABDOMINAL VISCERA.

During the progress of tuberculous consumption the mucous membrane of the alimentary canal rarely escapes disease. A distinguished pathologist observes, " Softening of the mucous membrane of the stomach, hyperæmia of the different portions of the intestines, ulceration of the small intestine, ac-companied in many instances by a development of tubercles, are all of such frequent occurrence in phthisis, that they may be fairly considered as con-stituent parts of the disease."* These morbid states of the alimentary canal generally occur sub-sequently to the pulmonary disease, although they occasionally appear to precede it; at least, I have observed the usual symptoms of diseased bowels some considerable time before those indicating dis-

* Andral, op. cit., vol. ii. p. 558.

ease of the lungs. This remark accords with the experience of Andral, who observes that " these lesions may either precede or follow the formation of tubercles in the lungs ; and in some cases the pulmonary and abdominal affections set in together." The stomach, the lower portion of the ileum, and the colon are the parts most frequently affected.

Morbid conditions of the stomach.—Inflammation of the mucous membrane of the stomach is not an unfrequent occurrence during the progress of consumption. It generally comes on at an advanced stage of the disease ; but I have occasionally found it present, in a slight degree, at its commencement. The symptoms are loss of appetite, thirst, nausea, and sometimes vomiting and epigastric pain on pressure. When the inflammation is situated in the anterior part of the stomach, the pain is generally much increased by pressure. Of one hundred and twenty-three phthisical patients observed by Louis, eight suffered from the present affection, and only one of this number was exempt from pain ;—in the others, a sensation of heat and of pain, much increased by pressure, was experienced in the epigastrium, and there was also a degree of resistance upon pressure, which was found to arise from enlargement of the liver.—Ulceration of the stomach is accompanied by nearly the same symptoms.

Another morbid condition of the stomach, the nature of which is not fully understood, is occasion-

ally met with in tuberculous subjects; its chief
symptoms are vomiting and pain.   Louis considers
it dependent upon softening and wasting of the
mucous membrane; but the experiments of Dr.
Carswell have clearly demonstrated that such softening of the coats of the stomach is a *post-mortem*
change produced by the action of the gastric fluid.
The red softening is essentially different in its nature,
and is the result of inflammation.   But, whatever be
the pathology of the gastric affection at present under consideration, it is very distressing to the patient,
and difficult to remedy.   According to the observations of Louis, it occurs from two to six months
before death ; but I have known it to exist for a much
longer period, and even long before any symptom
of pulmonary disease presented itself.   In one
young lady it existed for several years ; and it was
only within a few months of death that the pulmonary disease became evident.   The extent to which
the latter was found after death to have proceeded,
showed how long it had remained latent, masked
by the deranged condition of the stomach.   Another patient—a female, twenty-five years of age,
whose brother lately died of tuberculous consumption—has retained scarcely anything on her stomach
for upwards of two years, except a very little
water or toast-water ; every thing else is rejected
the moment it is swallowed.   The emaciation and
debility are very great.   She presents all the ex-

ternal characters of tuberculous cachexia, with a
short dry cough, and, if the affection of the stomach
do not previously prove fatal, will most probably
die of consumption at no very distant period. In
this case the pain in the epigastric region is not
great, even on pressure; but in some cases it is so
severe, and so entirely absorbs the patient's feelings
and attention, that without minute observation on
the part of the medical attendant, the pulmonary
disease may escape notice. In general, the stomach
can digest very little, and then only the lightest
food. Occasionally the appetite and powers of
digestion return for a time. This occurred in the
patient last mentioned; during a residence in the
country for several months in the summer, the stomach retained and digested light food well.

It becomes a matter of some moment, in a practical point of view, to distinguish the vomiting
which occurs in the course of consumption, (and
which is commonly attributed to the cough,) from
that which depends on a morbid state of the stomach. A little attention to the concomitant symptoms will generally enable us to make this distinction. When the vomiting is simply the consequence of the cough, we find no epigastric tenderness or pain; the appetite remains, and the
digestion, in the intervals of coughing, goes on
well: it frequently occurs at the commencement of
the disease. When, on the other hand it is the

result of a morbid condition of the stomach, it is generally preceded by loss of appetite and pain in the region of that organ—symptoms which continue and usually increase during the course of consumption : the period, also, at which vomiting first occurs in this case is generally late in the disease.

Enlargement of the stomach.—An increase in the size of the stomach has evidently an intimate connexion with consumption, as Louis found it in more than two-thirds of the cases which he examined ; while in two hundred and thirty subjects who died of other diseases, only two examples of enlargement presented themselves. It sometimes goes on till the organ acquires double or treble its usual volume, and descends so far into the abdomen as to be on a level with the spine of the pubis.

The other lesions observed in this organ do not appear to be necessarily connected with consumption, although their occurrence in the course of other chronic diseases is far less frequent. They consist of a thickened, reddened, mammellated, or ulcerated state of its mucous membrane.

The same lesions occur in the mucous membranes of the small and large intestines ; but in these they appear to have a more intimate relation to consumption.

Ulceration of the intestines.—Ulcers of the intestines, when first formed, are always small ; they occur most frequently in the lower portion of the ileum, and chiefly in that part opposite its attachment to the mesentery, where the glandulæ agminatæ are chiefly situated. These glands form their primary seat. In the large intestines the ulcerations occur irregularly. When the ulcerative process is once established, it often extends to the surrounding tissues; the neighbouring ulcers coalesce, and the mucous membrane is undermined or destroyed to a great extent. Louis found them spreading to the length of nine inches, and running quite round the colon. Perforation of the intestine, although a very rare occurrence in consumption, occasionally takes place.

The more early ulceration of the intestines occurs, the more rapid in general is the progress of the disease, because it is usually accompanied with intractable diarrhœa, which speedily wastes both the flesh and strength of the patient. Louis found tuberculous ulceration in the small intestines in *five-sixths* of the cases which he examined, and noticed it almost as frequently in the large intestines, the mucous membrane of which often presented other diseased appearances, being red, thickened, or softened in one-half of the cases; so that, of the whole number of phthisical cases examined by this physician, the large intestines were found in a healthy state through their whole extent in *three instances* only.

The mesenteric glands are very often found tuberculous, more especially in children. Papavoine found them so in one-half of the cases of tuberculous diseases of children; while in the cases of adults examined by Louis, they were tuberculous in something less than one-fourth only.

Disease of the liver.—The liver, in phthisis, presents one remarkable alteration of structure, which consists in its equable transformation into a fatty substance. This change appears to take place simultaneously over the whole organ, and to be intimately connected with the development of tubercles in other organs; for of forty-nine cases of this degeneration observed by Louis, forty-seven were phthisical; and of two hundred and thirty subjects who died from other diseases, it occurred in nine only, seven of whom had a few tubercles in the lungs. When far advanced, it soiled the scalpel and hands like common fat:—when the change existed in a less degree, its presence was detected by the impregnation of paper with fat, on a portion of the organ being enclosed in it and exposed to heat. This degeneration of the liver is marked by a pale fawn colour, diminished consistence, and increased bulk of the organ, which sometimes enlarges to double its usual size. The rapidity with which it takes place seems to depend almost entirely on the progress of consumption; for it has been found when this has run

M

through all its stages in fifty days. Its occurrence
is independent of the patient's age or strength of
constitution; sex, however, appears to have a decided influence, as of the forty-nine cases observed
by Louis, only ten were males. The causes which
conduce to this morbid change are very obscure:
affections of the duodenum, which Broussais
supposed to cause it, have been found by Louis to
have no influence in its production. It is yet more
remarkable that it is accompanied by no appreciable symptom except increase of bulk, and that
the functions of the organ seem to go on undis-
turbed. The liver occasionally contains tubercles,
particularly in children. A diseased state of the
liver appears more frequent in some localities than
in others. According to Desault, it is a very
common occurrence at Bordeaux; so much so, indeed, that he scarcely met with a case of consumption in which he did not find this organ affected
during life. " Je trouve constamment une obstruction bien marquée par dureté, et souvent douleur."*
This is certainly not the case in this country; for,
although a congested state of the liver is a frequent
attendant on phthisis, and often long precedes it,
still I believe that it does not often proceed to
such an extent as to form, during life, a perceptible
tumour in the abdomen; nor is the fatty degenera-

* Op. citat. p. 39.

tion of the liver so common in this country as in France.

Fistula in ano.—This affection has been frequently found in consumptive patients, and has been supposed to be connected with the disease. Although I have often met with it, I have been unable to trace any connexion between it and phthisis, further than its probable dependence on abdominal venous plethora, which so often precedes pulmonary consumption. Andral states that the result of his observations does not confirm the opinion of a connexion between the two diseases.

It occasionally happens that death occurs suddenly in the advanced state of the disease. The patient does not appear worse than he has been for some days, when, while sitting up, he suddenly falls back and expires. Examination after death does not always enable us to explain this sudden cessation of life. Louis gives two cases, in one of which œdema of the glottis appeared to be the cause ; and in the other, a rapid hepatization of a large portion of the lungs ; but neither of these pathological lesions could account for the sudden terminations to which I allude.

Among the causes of sudden death, *pulmonary hemorrhage* may be mentioned, as it is occasionally so profuse as to prove fatal in a few minutes. In such cases a considerable artery is opened by ulceration in the progress of the tuberculous disease.

I cannot conclude this chapter without expressing my obligations to M. Louis, the able author of the *Traité de la Phthisie*. We are so much indebted to this zealous and indefatigable physician for all our more precise knowledge of the morbid anatomy of consumption, that I think it due to him to acknowledge the great assistance I have derived from his researches on this part of the subject; and I beg to refer my readers for more full information to his work, as they will not only find therein the best account of the morbid anatomy and symptoms of the disease, but will moreover learn to admire, and perhaps to imitate, the indefatigable industry, the ardent zeal, and the scrupulous veracity of this very accurate and philosophical observer.*

* I am glad to find that Louis' work has been lately translated into English : *Pathological Researches on Phthisis*, by E. Ch. A. Louis, with Introduction, Notes, Additions, and an Essay on Treatment, by Charles Cowan, M.D., Bath.

CHAPTER VII.

TUBERCULOUS consumption is essentially a chronic disease, but the range of its duration is very considerable.

The following tables, extracted from the works of Bayle and Louis, give an accurate view of the duration of phthisis in three hundred and fourteen cases. In the first table the numbers of cases which came under the observation of each physician are given separately, in order to show how far they correspond.

The mean duration of phthisis calculated from this table is twenty-three months; but it will be observed that one hundred and sixty-two, or more than one-half of the cases, terminated in nine months, and the greatest proportion of these between the fourth and ninth months.

M. Andral's experience at La Charité led him to fix the average duration of the disease in that hospital at two years, which is very near the average deduced from the tables of Bayle and Louis; but, from an inspection of these tables, it is evident that much the larger proportion of cases die considerably within this period.

TABLE I.

Duration of Disease.	Number of Cases.		Number of Cases.		Total.
Months.	Louis.	Bayle.	Louis.	Bayle.	
1	1	1			
2	4	6	8 + 16 =		24
3	3	9			
4	5	12			
5	11	14	25 + 44 =		69
6	9	18			
7	9	18			
8	9	14	25 + 44 =		69
9	7	12			
10	4	8			
11	3	7	12 + 20 =		32
12	5	5			
13	2	6			
14	4	10	12 + 21 =		33
15	6	5			
16	0	3			
17	2	4	3 + 9 =		12
18	1	2			
19	1	2			
20	1	3			
21	0	6			
22	0	3	10 + 18 =		28
23	0	2			
24	8	2			
Years.					
3	6	6			
4	6	5	14 + 14 =		28
5	2	3			
6	0	1			
7	0	3			
8	0	1	1 + 9 =		10
9	0	3			
10	1	1			
12	2	1			
14	1	0	4 + 5 =		9
20	1	4			
40	0	0			
	114	200	114 + 200 =		314

The following table is constructed from the last. The numbers are reduced to proportions of one hundred, and placed so as to exhibit the law of mortality in phthisis. Supposing one hundred persons to be attacked with phthisis at the same time, the first column (1.) shows the number of deaths thàt will occur in three months, six months, &c.; the second column (2.) the number that are alive after the lapse of the same time; and the third column (3.) how many die in the various periods of the disease.

TABLE II.

Showing the rate of mortality in one hundred cases.

Time from the invasion of the disease.	1.	2.	3.	Periods of the disease.
	Dead.	Alive.	Die.	
Months.				Months.
3	8	92	8	From 1 to 3 inclusive
6	30	70	22	4 „ 6
9	52	48	22	7 „ 9
12	62	38	10	10 „ 12
15	72	28	10	13 „ 15
18	76	24	4	16 „ 18
24	85	15	9	19 „ 24
Years.				Years.
5	94	6	9	3 „ 5
10	97	3	3	6 „ 10
40	100	0	3	11 „ 40

It may be well for the reader to bear in mind that these tables are calculated from fatal cases which occurred in hospital practice.*

* I am indebted to my ingenious friend, Mr. William Farr, of Grafton-street, for constructing these two tables.

Various circumstances affect the duration of consumption: the age, sex, constitution, and external circumstances of the patient, such as occupation, the season of the year, climate, &c., have all, no doubt, their influence. Louis considers age as having little effect on the duration of phthisis, except in very acute cases, which are more frequent in early life. Although I cannot refer to cases with the numerical precision of that accurate physician, my own experience in this respect differs from that of M. Louis. He found the mortality greater within the first year among females than among males, in the proportion of forty-two to thirty; after this period the ratio of mortality as to time was the same in both sexes. In the upper ranks of society, where patients have all the advantages that the best regimen, change of air, and medical treatment can afford, the medium duration of phthisis is probably not much short of three years; under other circumstances it is less. It is melancholy to reflect that cures occur in so small a ratio that in estimating the duration of phthisis we cannot bring them into the calculation.

The duration of consumption is greatly influenced by the seasons, as appears by the following table, compiled from particulars given in Dr. Heberden's Bills of Mortality, which shows the disstribution of deaths from consumption, through the different months of the year in London.

TABLE III.

Months.	Deaths.	Months.	Deaths.
March	4634	November ..	3711
February	4527	June	3604
December ..	4516	October	3521
January	4363	July	3249
April	4227	September ..	2994
May	4043	August	2825

The months are placed according to the amount of mortality in each. The result accords with the common observation that the disease proves most fatal in the winter and spring. In the winter months the number of deaths is 13,406;—in the spring, 12,904; — in the autumn, 10,226; — in summer, 9678. Bayle's experience afforded him a different result, but his calculation was made on too small a number (250) to be of any value in determining the point.

CHAPTER VIII.

THE influence of age, of sex, of race, climate, &c., in disposing to tuberculous diseases generally, and the more decided effects of various occupations and modes of living in the production of consumption, form a very important subject of inquiry. It is, however, to be regretted that the materials which have hitherto been collected are still too scanty to enable us to enter into it so fully as its merits demand. But we trust that an inquiry of so much interest and utility will be soon elucidated by the more extended co-operation of numerous medical observers.

SECT. I.—PREVALENCE AND SITE OF TUBERCLES
AT THE DIFFERENT PERIODS OF LIFE.

Tubercles have been found in various organs at every age; they have even been discovered in the fœtus, most frequently in the form of transparent granulations, but occasionally in a soft-ened state.* Chaussier discovered miliary tubercles in the lungs of a fœtus which died at birth, and an encysted abscess, or rather vomica, in the lungs of another.† Oehler found the mesenteric glands swollen, hard, and of a fatty consistence, in the fœtuses not only of scrofulous mothers, but of others who did not present any appearance of scrofula.‡ Husson reported to the Paris Academy of Medicine the dissection of two infants, one eight days old, and the other still-born at the seventh month of pregnancy, both of which had tubercles in a state of suppuration; the former in the liver, the latter in the lungs.§ Billiard, who examined a great many infants at the Foundling Hospital of Paris, found tuberculous granulations of the peritoneum in an infant who died four days after birth; and in two still-born children he met with evident tuberculous disease of the mesenteric glands.‖ Although many other cases of the presence of tubercles in the fœtal state might be cited, still the fact that Velpeau and Breschet never observed

---

* Tubercles have been found in the placenta in several cases.

† Procès Verbale de la distribution des pris aux élèves sages-femmes de l'Hospice de la Maternité, an. 1812, p. 62.

‡ *Desormeaux*, Dict. de Médecine, vol. xv. art. *Œuf*, p. 402.

§ Ibid. p. 402.

‖ Traité des Maladies des Enfans nouveaux-nés et à la mamelle, p. 648.

them in the course of their researches,* and that
M. Guizot did not find a single example of tuberculous disease in four hundred new-born children
whom he examined, is sufficient to show that its
occurrence in the fœtus is comparatively rare.†

Tuberculous disease is frequently developed during infancy. Billiard found tuberculous granulations
of the spleen and liver in five infants whom he
examined at the Foundling Hospital; in two of the
cases there were also tubercles in the lungs : he
also found tubercles in the lungs of four children
in one year, all of whom appeared healthy at birth,
but gradually fell into a state of marasmus, and died
at the respective ages of one, two, three, and five
months, without presenting any of the symptoms
proper to the phthisis of adults.‡

We have not sufficient data to estimate the comparative frequency of tuberculous disease during
the first two years of life, yet we are well assured,
from observation, that it is not uncommon at this
early age. I have met with several cases of infants
dying of consumption within the first year, in whom
the lungs were not only extensively tuberculous,
but contained large caverns with all the characters
of those found in the lungs of adults. There is
reason to believe that the disease in infants is fre-

* Thesis, p. 10.
† Journal des Progrès, loc. cit.
‡ Op. citat.

quently overlooked from the symptoms being less evident than in more advanced life, and from the want of oral information. The expectoration also is rarely seen, and the cough often assumes the character of pertussis; so that the disease is not unfrequently mistaken for that or chronic catarrh.

After the second year of age, the great prevalence of tuberculous diseases has been remarked by many pathologists. M. Guersent, a physician of extensive experience attached to the Hôpital des Enfans Malades in Paris, where no patient is admitted below the first or above the sixteenth year, is of opinion that tubercles existed in two-thirds or even five-sixths of the bodies which he examined.[*] The researches of M. Lòmbard,[†] and more lately those of M. Papavoine,[‡] carried on in the same institution, have determined with great precision the frequency of tuberculous affections, and the differences in their prevalence at various periods of early life. From the records of deaths under fifteen years of age in the practice of the New Town Dispensary during two years, Dr. Alison is of opinion that the mortality from scrofulous diseases in the children of the lower orders in Edinburgh might be

* Clinical Reports, Journ. Hebdom. t. vii. p. 588.

† *Andral*, Anatomie Pathologique, Townsend and West's Translation, vol. i.

‡ Journal de Progrès.

estimated much higher than one-third of the whole deaths.*

The following table is calculated from six hundred and ninety-five examinations recorded by Papavoine and his colleagues. The bodies were examined with great care, and the tuberculous distinguished from the non-tuberculous for each year of age from the third to the fifteenth inclusive. It is, however, to be observed that in two-fifths of the cases the tuberculous disease was not the cause of death. It is probable that the numbers here given express with considerable accuracy the relative proportion of the tuberculous to the non-tuberculous that die in the hospital, and perhaps among the poor of Paris generally; but since the children admitted belong to the most indigent classes, and generally remain some time in the hospital, it may be supposed that the proportion of the tuberculous is exaggerated; as, however, Papavoine's observations do not include the deaths in the scrofulous wards, any error which may arise from these circumstances is probably obviated. To exhibit the influence of age on the production of tubercles the table was constructed by ascertaining the annual mortality in ten thousand individuals at each age, and setting down in opposite columns the proportions of the

* See his excellent paper, *Observations on the Pathology of Scrofulous Diseases*, in the first volume of the Trans. Med. Chir. Soc. Edinb.

tuberculous and the non-tuberculous determined from Papavoine. Ten thousand children are supposed to be alive at the beginning of each year. The first column gives the age; the second is calculated on the law of mortality in France, (Annuaire 1832, p. 83,) and shows the total number of deaths in the course of the year; the third shows the proportion of tuberculous, and the fourth the proportion of children not tuberculous, that die in the ten thousand. The fifth column gives the number of tuberculous in a hundred deaths.

TABLE IV.

Age.	Total deaths.	Tuberculous.	Non-tuberculous.	Tuberculous in one hundred deaths.
1	2630			0
2	1290	161*	1129*	12*
3	729	292	437	40
4	408	204	204	50
5	263	173	90	66
6	178	130	48	72
7	125	87	38	70
8	99	74	25	75
9	82	52	30	63
10	78	52	26	67
11	77	44	33	57
12	78	47.	31	60
13	80	60	20	75
14	84	56	28	66
15	89	47	42	52

* We have not sufficient data to establish the frequency of tubercles during the first two years of life; these numbers are given upon the authority of M. Lombard, according to whose researches, tubercles are found in only one-eighth of the children who die in the *Hôpital des Enfans Malades* at Paris, between the ages of one and two.

From an examination of this table, it would appear that age has more influence in determining tuberculous disease than all other appreciable causes taken together. The tendency to this process is five times more intense at one period of life than at another; it may, perhaps, be said that it is some hundreds of times more intense in the fourth year than at birth. The frequency of the disease is in no constant relation either to the mortality or the growth. Tubercles prevail most through the third, fourth, fifth, and sixth years, when the annual growth does not exceed one-tenth of the child's weight, and the mortality declines to nearly one in a hundred. Papavoine has fallen into an error in stating that tubercles are generally most frequent in those periods of life when the mortality is least. We find, by referring to the table, that the mortality is least (seventy-seven in the ten thousand) in the eleventh year, and forty-four only in the ten thousand die tuberculous : the mortality is much greater in the fourth year (four hundred and eight in the ten thousand), and so is the number of tuberculous (two hundred and four). The error originates in supposing that the number of the tuberculous is as the relation of the tuberculous to the non-tuberculous among the deaths. M. Andral says, after M. Lombard, that " tubercles are most prevalent from four to five: they appear in much greater quantities, and in a greater number of organs at once."* Now there is little doubt that the proportion of those who die tuberculous is at its maximum relatively to those who die without tubercles, about this period; but it is erroneous to suppose that a child five years of age is more liable to tubercles than a child of three:—indeed the contrary is the fact, for only one hundred and seventy-three aged five, and two hundred and ninety-two aged three years, are tuberculous in ten thousand. M. Andral, depending on the accuracy of these calculations, has been led into the error of concluding that every irritation or congestion is far more to be apprehended at this age than previously, inasmuch as it may be followed by the production of tubercles.

More than one-fourth (,27-100) of those who die from birth to puberty are affected with tuberculous disease ; yet it causes death in about one-sixth only of the cases. From the third year upwards these proportions are two-thirds and one-third.

The great prevalence of tuberculous diseases in early life, which the researches of these pathologists have demonstrated, is a subject highly deserving the attentive consideration of the physician. The mortality from these affections at this period is much greater than is generally believed ; at least, although I had long had occasion to remark

* Op. cit. vol. i. p. 528.

the frequency, I was not aware of the extensive prevalence of tubercles at so early an age, until I became acquainted with the results obtained by the French pathologists.

The practical inferences to be deduced from the facts above stated are sufficiently evident, and require little comment. They show the paramount importance of attending to the health of infants and children, particularly in scrofulous families. But I shall have occasion to revert to the consideration of this subject.

With the view of ascertaining the comparative prevalence of tuberculous disease at different periods of life, all the statistical reports which appeared worthy of attention have been examined. The results of the researches concerning the relative prevalence of phthisis at different ages above puberty, as shewn in the following tables, are so conclusive as to preclude the necessity of any comment. Table V. gives the numbers as they were found in the various works. Table VI., constructed from the preceding one, gives the absolute mortality from consumption,—the number of persons in the thousand who die at each age in the different places, and the average of the whole.

TABLE V.

Showing the mortality from consumption above the age of fifteen.

	Place of observation.	15 to 20	20 to 25	25 to 30	30 to 35	35 to 40	40 to 45	45 to 50	50 to 55	55 to 60	Above 60
1	Edinburgh..............	6	9	13	8	11	8	6	3	9	4
2	Berlin	18	28	27	27	39	29	20	32	39	53
3	Nottingham	42	73	76	46	51	28	20	11	5	6
4	Philadelphia	182	974		875		565		338		258
5	Chester	15	27		24		22		16		6
6	Carlisle	15	45		34		31		15		15
7	Paris—*Louis*............	11	39		33		23		12		5
8	Ditto—*Bayle*	10	23		23		21		15		8
9	Charleston..............	..	26		24		13		21		4
10	Ditto, Whites	..	14		17		10		3		3
11	Ditto, Blacks	..	15		13		9		3		3

TABLE VI.

Showing the proportion of one thousand deaths from consumption.

	Place of observation.	15 to 20	20 to 30	30 to 40	40 to 50	50 to 60	Above 60
1	Edinburgh................	78	285	245	182	157	52
2	Berlin	69	212	256	190	274	204
3	Nottingham	117	416	271	134	45	17
4	Philadelphia	59	305	275	178	106	81
5	Chester	136	245	218	200	145	54
6	Carlisle	97	290	219	200	97	97
7	Paris	92	325	275	192	100	42
8	Ditto...................	99	225	225	206	147	78
	Average of the above*	99	285	248	185	108	78

1. Reports of New Town Dispensary, three years, Edin. Journ. 1821-25.
2. Sussmilch Göttliche Ordnung.
3. Dr. Clark's Reports, 1806-10. Edin. Med. Journ.
4. American Journal of Med. Science, 1826-32.
5. Dr. Haygarth, Phil. Trans. vols. 64, 65.
6. Dr. Heysham on Mortality, &c. of Carlisle.
7. *Louis*, Traité de la Phthisie.
8. *Bayle*, Traité de la Phthisie Pulmonaire.

* In comparing this average, it must be borne in mind that the first column embraces a period of five years only, while the others comprise ten years.

The comparison of this general average with any of the separate observations will shew the correctness of the results by the similarity which it bears to many of them. It will be seen that, with one exception, all these instances, although collected under different circumstances of time, place, &c., agree in shewing the greatest number of deaths to occur between the age of twenty and thirty; the next in proportion between thirty and forty; the next between forty and fifty; the succeeding grade of mortality being sometimes placed between fifteen and twenty, at other times between fifty and sixty, or even above sixty. This remarkable agreement of all the places warrants the conclusion that, after the fifteenth year of age, fully one-half of the deaths from consumption occur between the twentieth and fortieth years of age, and that the mortality is about its maximum at thirty, and from that time gradually diminishes.

The researches of MM. Andral and Lombard have led them nearly to the same conclusions as those deduced from the preceding tables. The former considers that males are particularly subject to consumption between the ages of twenty-one and twenty-eight; while females seem to be more exposed to it before twenty.* The latter believes that females are most liable to tubercles between

* Op. cit. vol. i. p. 529.

their eighteenth and twentieth year, and males between twenty and twenty-five.*

The opinion of Hippocrates corresponds still more closely with the results obtained from these tables. That accurate observer fixed the age at which consumption most frequently occurs, between the eighteenth and thirty-fifth year.†

The site of tuberculous disease at the different periods of life is a circumstance deserving attention. The two following tables give a view of the localization of the disease in children and in adults. The first is from Papavoine's excellent memoir on tuberculous diseases, and is the result of *fifty* careful post-mortem examinations of children, made with the view of determining the relative frequency of tubercles in different organs.‡

TABLE VII.

Bronchial glands	49 times
Lungs	38 „
Cervical glands	26 „
Mesenteric glands	25 „
Spleen	20 „
Pleura	17 „
Liver	14 „
Small intestines	12 „
Peritoneum	9 „

* Op. cit. p. 29.
† Coac. Progn. 439.
‡ Journal de Progrès des Sciences Médicales, t. ii. p. 93.

Large intestines	9 times
Brain	5 „
Cerebellum	3 „
Membranes of the brain	3 „
Pericardium	„
Kidneys	2 „
Stomach	1 „
Pancreas	1 „
Vertebræ, radius, tibia	1 „

A comparison of this with the result of Louis's observations, as given in the following table referring to persons above the age of fifteen, who died of consumption, will show the relative occurrence of tubercles in different organs in the two periods of life.*

TABLE VIII.

Small intestines	about $\frac{1}{4}$
Large intestines	„ $\frac{1}{5}$
Mesenteric glands	„ $\frac{1}{4}$
Cervical glands	„ $\frac{1}{10}$
Lumbar glands	„ $\frac{1}{12}$
Prostate	„ $\frac{1}{13}$
Spleen	„ $\frac{1}{14}$
Ovaries	„ $\frac{1}{20}$
Kidneys	„ $\frac{1}{60}$

SECT. II.—THE INFLUENCE OF SEX IN DETERMINING THE PREVALENCE OF CONSUMPTION.

It has generally been believed that consumption is more prevalent among females than among males;

* *Louis*, Op. cit. Rapport, pp. 4, 5.

but as the Paris Reports have been the chief sources
from which statistical information on this subject
has been obtained, it is evident that the law of
comparative mortality from phthisis which results
from the observations hitherto made there, is not
applicable to the comparative mortality from the disease in other places. It will be seen by the following table that in this respect Paris forms a remarkable exception to the other places for which we have
been able to collect materials for calculations.

TABLE IX.

	Place.	Males.	Females.	Males.	Fe-males.
1	Hamburgh	555	445	10 to	8·7
2	Rouen Hospital.	55	44	10 to	8·6
3	Naples Hospital..........	382	315	10 to	8·2
4	New York	1584	1370	10 to	8·6
5	Geneva	71	62	10 to	8·7
6	Berlin	328	292	10 to	8·8
7	Sweden	2088	1860	10 to	8·9
8	Ditto	3054	3103	10 to	10·4
9	Berlin..................	560	655	10 to	11·6
10	Blacks, New York........	47	58	10 to	12·3
11	Paris	2219	2970	10 to	13·3
12	Ditto	3965	5579	10 to	14·3
13	Berlin, boys and girls	363	567	10 to	15·6

1. *Julius Nachrichten* ueber die Hamburgischen Krankenhaüser, 1829
2. *Hellis*, Clin. Méd. de l'Hôtel Dieu de Rouen, 1825.
3. *Renzi*, Topog. Med. di Napoli.
4. New York Med. and Phys. Register.
5. Chisholm on the Climate and Diseases of Tropical Countries.
6. Sussmilch Göttliche Ordnung.
7. Kön Swenska Vetanskaps Hand. 1801. Nicandar.
8. Ditto, quoted from Marshall's Statistics of the British Empire.
9. Neue Berliner Monat Schrift, 1809, p. 225.
10. New York Med. and Phys. Register.
11. Conseil de Salubrité.
12. *Chabrol*, Statistique de la Ville de Paris.
13. Neue Berliner Monat Schrift, 1809, p. 225.

The two first columns in the preceding table give the facts as they were found ; the two last columns show the relative deaths, ten being taken for the number of males.

Any conclusion which might be drawn from this table can only be considered an approximation to the truth, and is liable to error, from our neither knowing the relative number of the sexes alive in each place, their relative deaths from other diseases, nor their relative admissions into the hospitals referred to. The smallness of the numbers also allows any accidental circumstances to modify the result. In noticing the observations more particularly, I shall refer to the number of each place.

Nos. 1 *to* 7.—The constant equal relation of the first seven numbers is certainly most remarkable, and appears to warrant the conclusion that, for every eight or nine females, ten males die phthisical, which is very nearly the relative number of the sexes : it therefore goes far to prove that the sexes are equally subject to consumption. *Nos.* 8 *and* 9, do not materially affect the preceding conclusion, as the preponderance of deaths among the females would probably be counterbalanced by more extended observations. *No.* 10, referring to the Blacks, is of little value on account of the small number of cases to which it refers, and by our ignorance of the relation of the sexes in a Black population. *No.* 13, is a very curious observation ; it does not, however, apply to the general calculation, as it refers to children only. If it be correct, it would show that, in childhood, consumption is much more frequent among females than among males, at Berlin. *Nos.* 11 *and* 12 are in direct contradiction to the first seven observations, and differ widely from Nos. 8 and 9, but approach 13 rather closely. They would show that in Paris the disease is more prevalent among females than among males by about one-fifth ; and it is worthy of remark that other observations made there have led to the same conclusion. M. Lepelletier found that the number of phthisical females admitted into the hospitals of Paris were in relation to the males as five to three. We have no statistical reports in this country on a sufficiently extended scale, to enable us to institute a comparison on this subject between England and other countries.

SECT. III.—THE INFLUENCE OF CERTAIN OCCU-
PATIONS IN INDUCING CONSUMPTION.

Although from an early period medical writers have noticed the influence of certain occupations in producing[1] pulmonary disease, it is only of late years that their attention has been more particularly directed to this very important subject. Those

trades which expose the workmen to an atmosphere
loaded with pulverulent bodies or charged with
gaseous substances of an irritating quality, and
sedentary occupations of all kinds, are believed to
exert a deleterious action on the respiratory organs,
and to induce pulmonary consumption; while, on
the contrary, occupations which require constant
exercise in the open air are as generally considered
to afford protection against the disease.

Up to a very recent period, writers on this subject contented themselves with giving the results of
their observation in a general manner; but of late
attempts have been made to determine the relative
effect of different occupations by numerical tables.
Of this kind are the observations of M. Benoiston de
Chateauneuf, published in the Annales d'Hygiène,
and the more recent researches of M. Lombard,
recorded in the same journal. In order, by this
method, to ascertain with precision to what extent
consumption is produced by the circumstances in
which individuals are placed by particular pursuits,
it would be necessary to ascertain the whole number of persons engaged in any particular pursuit,
the total number of deaths from all diseases, the
number of deaths from consumption, and, lastly,
the results compared with the mortality of the population of the place generally. This process
would require to be repeated for each trade. Possessed of such data upon a sufficiently extensive

scale, we might arrive at accurate conclusions
respecting the influence of occupation in the production of this disease ; and having established
the aggregate effect of the circumstances connected
with the exercise of any particular trade, we might,
by a careful study of all such circumstances taken
separately, refer each to its proper place in the
scale of causes, and determine its positive effect.

Researches of this kind, if carefully conducted,
could not fail to lead to valuable practical results,
by showing what alteration of circumstances might
render any particular trade more salubrious. The
materials, however, for such calculations do not
exist, although they are essentially necessary to
enable us to speak with precision on a question of
so much importance. The most complete information which we at present possess on the subject is
contained in the paper of M. Lombard already referred to ; but unfortunately the calculations adduced by him to show the prevalence of consumption
in the different trades at Geneva, although very
valuable in enabling us to approximate to the truth,
are defective, inasmuch as the number of persons
engaged in each trade is not stated. In consequence
of this defect it is impossible to ascertain the absolute frequency of consumption, and we can only determine its prevalence in relation to the total mortality
in each trade, which may of course vary from
many causes ; and trades the most unhealthy in other

respects may appear the most healthy in regard to consumption. Our other sources of information are still more deficient in the essential elements of such calculations, so that in the present state of the subject we are unable to determine by numbers the relative influence of trades, and must therefore endeavour to arrive at the most probable conclusions by reasoning upon such general observations as we possess.

All the agencies enumerated by authors may be reduced to two classes, the first embracing those which act as local irritants to the lungs; the second, those which exert an injurious effect on the whole economy. These two classes are so distinct in their nature that the evidence of their influence, and the consideration of the manner in which they lead to pulmonary disease, might, with great propriety, be separately investigated, if they were not so frequently combined.

The occupations which have been noticed by various authors as exerting a direct influence in irritating the respiratory organs and inducing pulmonary consumption, comprise a large proportion of our mechanics; such as stone-masons, miners, coal-heavers, flax-dressers, brass and steel-polishers, metal-grinders, needle-pointers, and many others who are exposed during their labours to the inhalation of an atmosphere charged with irritating particles.

Dr. Alison states that there is hardly an instance of a mason, regularly employed in hewing stones in Edinburgh, living free from phthisical symptoms to the age of fifty.* Mr. Thackrah remarks that masons are generally intemperate; they are exposed to the vicissitudes of the weather, to great bodily exertion, and to the inhalation of fine particles of sand, dust, and powdered stone : they are subject to chronic inflammation of the bronchial membrane and to pains of the limbs, and generally die before the age of forty.† Miners, as we learn from the same author, particularly while cutting through sandstone, are much exposed to the inhalation of dust; but they also take large quantities of ardent spirits, and seldom attain the age of forty. Dr. Forbes also states that an immense proportion of the miners in Cornwall are destroyed by chronic bronchitis; one of the principal, though by no means the sole cause of which he considers to be the inhalation of dust.‡ Wepfer remarked the destruction of the miners in his time employed in cutting

---

* Op. citat.

† On the Effects of Arts, Trades, and Professions, &c. on Health and Longevity. By C. Turner Thackrah, Esq.

‡ Translation of Laennec, second edition, p. 137. For extensive statistical researches respecting the health of this class of men, see an admirable essay on the Medical Topography of the Land's End, by Dr. Forbes, in the second volume of the Trans. of the Provincial Med. and Surg. Association.

millstones from the mines of Waldschut on the Rhine, where all the men are said to have become consumptive.*

The inhalation of silex in a minute state of division is shown by Benoiston de Chateauneuf and by M. Clozier to be equally pernicious. The latter, speaking of the workmen in the quarries of St. Roch, says, " Quelque forts et robustes que soient ces ouvriers, les uns plutôt, les autres plus tard, mais ordinairement avant quarante ans, sont attaqués d'abord d'une toux sèche," &c. and few pass the age of forty.† The pernicious effects of this labour are so well known that the disease is commonly called " La Maladie de St. Roch." The evidence of Chateauneuf on this point is even more conclusive :— the entire population of the small commune of Meusnes has been for the last hundred years exclusively employed in the manufacture of gun-flints ; during this period the mortality has increased to a frightful extent, and the mean duration of life has diminished in proportion.

The inhalation of metallic particles appears also to be highly injurious to the respiratory organs, and is perhaps as destructive of life. The pernicious effects of needle-pointing were long since described by Dr. Johnstone of Worcester ;‡ and Thackrah

* Observ. de capitis affect.
† *Le Blanc,* Œuvres Chirurgicales, vol. i. p. 585.
‡ Memoirs of Med. Soc. Lond. vol. v.

notices the operation of dry-filing cast-iron as most
injurious to the workmen. The mouth and nose
are blackened; the lining membrane of the nostrils,
where the annoyance is first felt, discharges co-
piously; the fauces become preternaturally dry, and
respiration is difficult: habitual cough succeeds, accompanied with derangement of the digestive organs
and morning vomiting; and the common termination is bronchial disease, and no doubt often tuberculous consumption: while, on the other hand,
dealers in old iron, whose clothes are covered with
a thick brown layer of metallic dust, suffer no inconvenience. Thackrah attributes the mortality of
the filers to the greater irritation of the mucous
membranes of the respiratory organs produced by
the angular particles of steel. The filers are remarkably short-lived; in the two principal machine
manufactories at Leeds there were only two filers of
the age of forty-eight. The men of these establishments are not intemperate; nor can their shortness
of life be attributed to anything but their employment. But the history of the grinders of Sheffield,
recorded by Dr. Knight, affords one of the most
striking examples of the pernicious influence of the
inhalation of mechanical irritants with which we
are acquainted; and the deleterious effect of such
inhalation is further illustrated by the difference
between the health of the dry and that of the
wet grinders. The grinders " altogether amount
to about two thousand five hundred; of this

number one hundred and fifty, namely eighty men
and seventy boys, are fork-grinders : these grind
dry, and die from twenty-eight to thirty-two years
of age. The razor-grinders grind both wet and dry,
and they die from forty to forty-five years of age.
The table-knife-grinders work on wet stones, and
they live to betwixt forty and fifty years of age."*
Dr. Knight is of opinion that the grit-dust is not
only the most copious, but also the most injurious
part of what is inhaled by the grinders. On comparing the diseases of these men with that of the
other mechanics in Sheffield, he found that of two
hundred and fifty grinders, one hundred and fifty-
four laboured under disease of the chest; while
only fifty-six were similarly affected in the same
number of workmen engaged in other trades. On
examining the respective ages of grinders and other
workmen, he obtained the following results :—

Age.	Grinders.	Other workmen.
Above 30	124	140
35	83	118
40	40	92
45	24	70
50	10	56
55	4	34
60	1	19
	286	529†

* North of England Med. and Surg. Journal, vol. i. p. 86.

† The disease which thus embitters the life of the grinder, and
ultimately destroys him when he has scarcely attained one half
the ordinary age of man, is generally denominated *grinders'
asthma*, and often, from its great fatality, *grinders' rot.*

Many more instances might be adduced to show the pernicious effects of mechanical irritants applied to the mucous membrane of the respiratory organs in producing fatal disease of the lungs; but the account of the grinders and flint-cutters which has just been given, is so conclusive that it is unnecessary to enter more fully into this part of our subject. There are, however, other circumstances in the history of these cases of chronic bronchial disease which deserve particular consideration, in addition to the question of pulmonary irritation which we have just discussed. In almost every instance the sufferers are exposed to causes fully adequate to the production of the tuberculous cachexia; they pass much of their time in a confined deteriorated atmosphere, often in a sedentary posture unfavourable to the free action of the respiratory organs; many of them are much exposed to the vicissitudes of the weather, and the majority are addicted to the use of ardent spirits.

The influence of confined and deteriorated atmosphere is shown in a remarkable manner in the fork-grinders resident in the town of Sheffield, and those employed in the same occupation in the country. The former die, as has been stated, between the ages of twenty-eight and thirty-two; the latter generally attain the age of forty. In both cases the exposure to mechanical irritation is the same, and the habits of the grinders in and out of Sheffield

o

do not differ; but the rooms in which the country workmen carry on their occupation are much better ventilated.

Persons employed in many other manufactories suffer in the same manner, but in a less degree. Feather-dressers and brush-makers, according to Chateauneuf, are confined to close apartments, and generally work in a sitting posture. In the former trade the deaths from pulmonary disease amount to 11·47 in the hundred, and in the latter to 7·76. Thackrah observes that in such trades the digestive organs are even sooner disordered than those of respiration. The process of flock-dressing appears to be most pernicious in this respect. " The subsequent sieving and examining of flocks produces great dust, and decidedly injures both respiration and digestion. In proportion to the degree and continuance of this deleterious agent is the head affected, the appetite reduced, respiration impeded, cough, and finally bronchial or tubercular consumption produced." " Dressers of flax and persons in the dusty rooms of the mills," he continues, " are generally unhealthy. They are subject to indigestion, morning vomiting, chronic inflammation of the bronchial membrane, inflammation of the lungs, and pulmonary consumption."* In all these cases the effect of the causes acting on

Op. cit. pp. 26 and 71.

the general system is made evident by the prominent place which disordered digestion, &c. hold among the symptoms enumerated. When disease is produced by bronchial irritation alone, these symptoms are not present, or occur only at a late period of the disease.

With respect to the nature of the pulmonary disease induced by the inhalation of mechanical irritants, of which the hard impalpable kind, according to the researches of Lombard, are the most injurious, our information is still very defective. It is surprising, indeed, how few accurate examinations have been made and recorded of individuals dying under the circumstances described. The symptoms are so similar to those of tuberculous phthisis, and are no doubt so often connected with it, that we shall only be able to state how far the mechanical irritation of the bronchial membrane contributes to the development of tuberculous disease, when we have a considerable series of well-conducted postmortem examinations of mechanics employed in the operations referred to, and of others who are engaged in similar occupations without being at the same time exposed to the action of mechanical irritants on the organs of respiration. That sufficient disease is induced to destroy life, with fearful rapidity, and to an immense extent, is fully established ; but I have no doubt that in many cases tuberculous disease has no share in it. My opinion on this point will, I apprehend, be confirmed by the following summary of all the morbid inspections of the disease which I have been able to collect.

In the cases of the stone-masons of Edinburgh, reported by Dr. Alison, he enumerates the following as the appearances generally observed : " portions of the lungs hardened and condensed, others in a soft pulpy state, nearly resembling the ordinary texture of the spleen, and others loaded with effused serum, with much adhesion of the pleuræ and much effusion into the bronchi."* These are certainly not the appearances presented by tuberculous disease of the lungs ; and I quite agree with Dr. Alison that they were the consequence of inflammation.

Dr. Hastings, in his excellent work on Bronchitis, has recorded the examination of three leather-dressers, (his eighth, tenth, and eleventh cases,) who died from pulmonary disease excited by the inhalation of dust. In the first of these cases, the lungs were more solid than natural ; the mucous membrane of the bronchi much inflamed, thickened, and containing several extensive superficial ulcers ; the bronchi filled with purulent fluid mixed with blood ; no tubercles were found. In the next case, the mucous membrane of the trachea and bronchi was highly inflamed and ulcerated ; the air-cells were filled with mucus mixed with pus ; the lungs strongly

Op. cit. p. 372.

adherent over the whole surface, their substance was
much gorged with blood; no tubercles. In these
cases, the heart was enlarged. In the third case, the
bronchial membrane was thickened and ulcerated;
there were many tubercles in both lungs, some
of them in a state of suppuration. Dr. Knight has
recently favoured me with an account of two cases
which have occurred to him since the publication of
his valuable paper in the North of England Medical
Journal.* Dr. Knight's first case was that of a fork-
grinder, who died July 31st, 1831, at the age of
thirty-eight, and had lost two brothers, also grinders,
at the respective ages of twenty-four, and twenty-
eight years. The examination disclosed the following appearances : extensive adhesion of the pleuræ,
especially on the right side; tubercles mostly in a
crude state in both lungs ; in the superior posterior
part of the left lung was a mass of the appearance
and consistence of cartilage, and of the size of a
pigeon's egg; upper part of the right lung indurated ; numerous ulcers in the bronchial membrane,
particularly of this lung, over which the adhesion
of the pleura was most extensive and firm. Several
bronchial glands were enlarged and indurated; the
larynx and trachea were free from disease; heart of

* It is gratifying to learn that the objections to *post-mortem*
examinations, which have hitherto been almost insurmountable, are
beginning to abate ; and no doubt the subject will now be fully
investigated.

natural size. The immediate cause of this man's
death was acute inflammation of the peritoneum and
pericardium, presenting the usual appearances. The
second case was a scissor-grinder, aged forty-seven,
of a scrofulous habit, very temperate and industrious.
He had for many years laboured under cough, at
times dry, and at others accompanied with copious
muco-purulent expectoration. The following appearances were observed on examination forty-eight
hours after death : adhesions to a considerable extent between the pleuræ; upper part of both lungs
emphysematous, particularly the right, which was
gorged with blood to the extent of a large orange,
but not indurated, immediately below the emphysematous portion. In the same lung were a large
cretaceous mass inclosed in a cartilaginous cyst, and
many tubercles in an indurated state. The left lung
likewise contained many small hard tubercles, and
at its posterior part a small collection of pus in a
cartilaginous cyst. The bronchial glands were enlarged ; the bronchial membrane was red, softened,
and covered with pus and blood. Heart adherent
to pericardium; many of the mesenteric glands
enlarged and of cretaceous consistence; mucous
membrane of the stomach extremely vascular and
softened, and thickly covered with red blood. The
patient had vomited a pint of fluid blood a few
hours before death.

Such, I apprehend, are the appearances which

will be generally found in these cases, viz., vascular congestion and ulceration of the bronchial membrane, congestion or induration of the pulmonary substance, and adhesions of the pleuræ; in many, complicated with emphysema, tubercles, and enlarged heart. The mechanical irritation of the respiratory organs, the sedentary habits and constrained position of the workman, the impure air which he breathes, and his usual habits of life, are abundantly sufficient to account for all these morbid changes; the mechanical irritation alone is not sufficient to produce them. In two of Dr. Hastings' cases, wherein mechanical irritation of the bronchial membrane had been maintained for many years together, extensive disorganization was thereby produced, and death caused without the formation of a single tubercle. In regard to Dr. Knight's second case, it deserves remark that the grinder was originally of the tuberculous constitution, and that he had passed the ordinary term of a grinder's life; and notwithstanding the constant irritation kept up in the lungs by his occupation, nature had made considerable advances to effect a cure of the tuberculous disease. It has already been observed, with respect to Dr. Alison's cases of the stone-masons in Edinburgh, whose occupation is constantly carried on in the open air, that no tubercles were found in the lungs. But there can be no doubt that a very considerable proportion of such mechanics will be found to have real tuberculous disease; as when a disposition to it exists, nothing is more likely to prove an exciting cause than the perpetual irritation produced by the inhalation of mechanical particles.

I shall now notice some circumstances which affect the general health of labourers, and thereby induce tuberculous cachexia. Among these none operate more injuriously in disposing to this morbid state than the deficient bodily exercise, and the want of pure air, which are generally united with sedentary occupations. Shoemakers, tailors, weavers, and dress-makers, may be cited among those who suffer most from these causes. Their sedentary employment, the constrained posture which it requires, and the crowded and ill-ventilated apartments in which it is generally carried on, are eminently calculated to prevent the free exercise of the respiratory organs, to diminish the powers of the circulation, to impair the nutritive function, and produce a corresponding depression of nervous energy. Their habits also are frequently careless and irregular; they adopt little precaution against the vicissitudes of temperature, and expose themselves to the influence of cold and damp, and too often to the evils arising from dram-drinking, and to those other causes which are most likely to produce congestions, fevers, and inflammations. If the female dress-makers, and other females employed in similar occupations, are exempted from some of these causes, the almost total privation of exercise, the late hours and long duration of their work are more than sufficient to injure, if not destroy, their health in a few years.

Now in these circumstances we find the conditions most favourable to the development of the general tuberculous diathesis, as well as those which have a peculiar influence in promoting its manifestation in the lungs. The effect of sedentary habits in all classes and conditions of society is in my opinion most pernicious ; and there is perhaps no cause, not even excepting hereditary predisposition, which exerts such a decided influence in the production of consumption, as the privation of fresh air and free exercise. Indeed, the result of my inquiries leads to the conviction that sedentary habits are among the most powerful causes of tuberculous disease, and that they operate in the higher classes as the principal cause of its greater frequency among females. In this rank of society we find the mortality from consumption below the average, almost all the active causes of the disease being removed. Lombard calculated that the disease is only one half as prevalent among persons in easy circumstances as it is among the great bulk of the population.

There are certain occupations which are generally considered unfavourable to the occurrence of consumption ; those of seamen, butchers, and tanners hold the first rank. Various reasons have been

adduced to account for this exemption. I have no
doubt that it is chiefly attributable to the free and
regular exercise in the open air which they enjoy.*

The facts which have been adduced in this section,
although they are, I admit, imperfect, may nevertheless lead to useful practical results. They not
only open an interesting field of observation and
inquiry, but suggest measures for improving the
health and condition of society, which are simple,
and in many cases available. We can only expect
to see a decided diminution of disease among the
industrious artisans of this country, when their work-
shops and apartments are more spacious and better
ventilated, when their physical powers are less
exposed to the depressing influence of variable
temperature, when they take more exercise in the
open air, pay more regard to cleanliness, and
cease to seek excitement in the pernicious habit
of spirit-drinking.

* I beg to refer the reader who is desirous of more minute information, to the writings of Dr. Beddoes, who has collected a
considerable body of evidence on the subject of this section ; to
Mr. Thackrah's valuable work on the Effects of Trades ; to Dr.
Forbes's able Memoir in the Transactions of the Provincial Medical
and Surgical Association ; to the excellent articles of Benoiston
de Chateauneuf, and our friend Dr. Lombard of Geneva, in the
Annales d'Hygiène ; and of Dr. Knight and Dr. Kay, in the North
of England Medical Journal.

SECT. IV.—THE INFLUENCE OF CLIMATE IN THE
PRODUCTION OF CONSUMPTION.

Our information respecting the influence of
climate in the production of tuberculous disease
is still very imperfect, and its operation as a predisposing and exciting cause has not been sufficiently
discriminated.

A cold, damp, and variable climate, such as that
of this country, not only gives the predisposition to
the disease, but becomes its exciting cause, and determines in an especial manner its local manifestation
in the lungs. Sir Alexander Crichton states that
" consumption is infinitely more frequent in Great
Britain and Ireland, in comparison of their population, than in the northern parts of Russia; yet the
climate of Russia is in general infinitely colder and
ruder than ours. The scrofulous or strumous constitution is more common in the northern and middle
governments of Russia than in England, and com-
mits greater ravages and disfiguration than are ever
witnessed in this country. Great Britain no where
exhibits such dreadful effects of scrofula as Russia
does; but in that empire its attacks are mostly confined to the external set of glands, to the face, the
eyes, and throat, and to the bones, especially those
of the extremities; the lungs suffer rarely, except
in public schools, and among those who adopt the

European dress and fashions."* There are, however, circumstances which must be taken into account in estimating the influence of the respective
climates of Russia and England ; the Russians clothe
themselves more warmly, and take greater precautions against the severity of the climate than the
English ; on the other hand, their poorer classes are
worse fed, black sourish rye-bread and vegetables
being their chief nourishment. The occupations also
of the Russians are for the most part in the open
air ; whereas a large proportion of the labouring
classes in England are employed in manufactories,
in which they are shut up for the greater part of the
day in a confined and deteriorated atmosphere.

Great heat appears to have a powerful effect in
predisposing to tuberculous disease. The general
constitution of the inhabitants of very hot countries,
as the Malays and Negroes, may be cited in confirm-
ation of this opinion, as both these races are well
known to be much more subject to tuberculous
disease than Europeans, when exposed to the same
causes. I shall adduce further proof of this in
the subjoined tables, containing a statistical account
of the prevalence of phthisis in different countries.

The facts relating to the prevalence of consumption in different nations, which I have been able to
collect from their statistical documents, are so dis-

* Pract. Obs. on Pulmonary Consumption, p. 50, &c.

crepant that no positive conclusion can be drawn from them to shew the effect of climate in producing the tuberculous diathesis. In this state of the subject I had recourse to the Records of the British army, as a source from which sufficient information might be collected to enable me to come to a probable conclusion. To avoid the errors which are liable to arise from calculations founded on one series of observations, two tables were constructed from different data bearing on the same subject. One was formed from the records of single regiments during the period of their foreign service ; the other table was calculated from the mortality in large bodies of troops on the different stations, during a period varying from three to seven years. This is stated to shew that some confidence may be placed in the subjoined table, as the ultimate result of a great number of distinct observations. The mortality of London is given as a point of comparison. But in comparing the mortality of the metropolis with that of the army, it must be kept in mind that the former includes the deaths at all ages, whereas in the army the ages generally vary from twenty to fifty.

The mortality from consumption is greater in the West Indies than any other station, and least at the Cape of Good Hope and the East Indies. The great prevalence of consumption in the West Indies I consider one of the most remarkable results of

my researches ; it confirms in a striking manner
the opinion I gave in another work on the injurious
effects of that climate on consumptive patients sent
there from this country.* The general mortality is
also greater in the West Indies than on any other
station, with the exception of the west coast of
Africa.†

* Influence of Climate, p. 115. &c.

† I avail myself of this opportunity to express my acknow-
ledgements to Sir James M'Gregor, Director General of the
Army Medical Department, and Sir William Burnett, Physician
General of the Navy, to whose kindness I am indebted for the
facilities afforded of examining the valuable collection of journals
and reports of the medical officers of the army and navy.

TABLE X.

Showing the effect of climate in determining the prevalence of consumption among the troops.

Stations where troops were employed.	Tables.	Yearly deaths from all diseases in every 1,000 men.	Yearly deaths from Phthisis in every 1,000 men.	Average mortality in 1,000 men.	
				From all diseases.	From consumption.
East Indies and New South Wales	1st table 2d table	76.9 38.2	.6 1.5	57.5	1.0
Cape of Good Hope	1st table 2d table	16.0 13.0	1.4 1.8	14.5	1.6
West coast of Africa	2d table			144.5	1.7
Mauritius	1st table 2d table	30.4 26.0	4.1 2.4	28.2	3.2
West Indies, Europeans	1st table 2d table	70.0 90.6	5.7 4.1	80.3	4.9
West Indies, Negroes	1st table 2d table	27.0 26.3	17.2 10.2	26.6	13.7
Bermudas	2d table			12.4	2.3
Canadas & Nova Scotia	1st table 2d table	12.5 11.9	3.5 3.4	12.2	3.4
Malta	1st table 2d table	15.1 14.4	2.4 2.8	14.7	2.6
Gibraltar	1st table 2d table	17.2 9.0	2.9 1.9	13.1	2.4
Ionian Islands	1st table 2d table	15.9 27.4	2.2 2.1	26.6	2.1
Malta, Gibraltar, Portugal, & Ionian Islands	1st table			24.2	1.6
City of London	1820 to 1830			19.0	6.2

I am far from placing implicit confidence on the results of the preceding table; they are only to be regarded as approximations to the truth. The whole subject of medical statistics is still in its infancy. To determine the influence of climate, we would require accurate information on the prevalence, not only of consumption, but also of all the forms in which the tuberculous diathesis manifests itself among the inhabitants; for the influence of any climate in producing this diathesis cannot be estimated from tables illustrating the prevalence of one form of the disease among strangers, who, of course, brought with them that disposition to the disease. It may, therefore, seem that I have arrived too hastily at the conclusion that tuberculous diseases are very prevalent among the natives of warm climates, more particularly the Negro race. I have, however, been led to it by considering their physical peculiarities, by the general character of their diseases, and by the fact that when these people are removed to Europe, the diathesis manifests itself rapidly in its most characteristic form of crude tubercles, not in the lungs merely, but simultaneously in almost every organ of the body.

The following table has been compiled from the Army Medical Records, for the purpose of determining the relative prevalence of phthisis and other diseases of the lungs among the Blacks and Europeans in the West Indies.

TABLE XI.

Shewing the relative mortality from consumption, &c. among the Blacks and Whites of the West Indian army, for eight years—1822 to 1829.

	Deaths from all diseases.	Deaths from Phthisis.	Deaths from other pulmonary diseases.
Whites........	2275	177	100
Blacks	555	158	105

By our calculations from the above table, we find that in every thousand deaths among the Whites, one hundred and twenty, or little more than one-eighth, are from pulmonic diseases ; while in every thousand deaths among the Blacks, four hundred and seventy-two, or nearly one-half, are caused by pulmonic diseases.

The following table has been constructed to show that phthisis is not only relatively but absolutely more prevalent among the natives than among Europeans in the East Indies: it has been compiled from Mr. Marshall's Medical Topography of Ceylon.

TABLE XII.

	Europeans.	Malays.	Caffres.	Indians.
Total deaths in 1000 persons during one year	142	36	49	45
Deaths from phthisis in 1000 persons during one year ..	.6	2.0	7.0	2.6
Deaths from phthisis in 1000 deaths from all diseases ..	4.3	58	146	59

SECT. V. INCREASE OR DECREASE OF CON-
SUMPTION.

As various opinions are entertained respecting
the increase or decrease of consumption in this
country, the following table has been constructed
with the view of determining this point.

TABLE XIII.

*Shewing the mortality from consumption in London during
the 18th and 19th centuries.*

Population within the Bills of Mortality, 1700 to 1821.		Average yearly number of deaths.			Number of yearly deaths in every 1000.		Number of deaths from consumption in every 1000 deaths from all diseases.
		1700 to 1830.	From all diseases.	From consumption.	From all diseases.	From consumption.	
1700	665,200	1700–10	20,943	3055	31	4	145
1750	653,900	1750–60	20,349	4373	31	6⅔	214
1801	777,000	1800–10	18,890	4979	24	6	263
1811	888,000	1810–20	19,061	5491	21	6⅙	288
1821	1,050,500	1820–30	20,679	6552	19	6⅕	316

This table is constructed from data contained in
Mr. Marshall's work, ' *On the Statistics, Mortality,
&c. of the Metropolis.*' It appears that from 1700
to 1750 the deaths from consumption increased from
4 to 6 in every 1000 of the population, and that
since the last period they have remained stationary.

The opinion entertained by some authors that consumption has increased since 1750 originates in the error of taking its *relative* mortality, as compared with that from all diseases, instead of its *absolute* mortality in reference to the population. It now appears to constitute *one-third* of the whole mortality. This relative increase does not arise from the increase of consumption, but depends on the diminished mortality from other diseases; the causes which have had so beneficial an influence in diminishing the number of deaths from them having produced no sensible effect on that from consumption. These calculations, however, are only to be considered as approximations to the truth; our bills of mortality must be kept in a very different manner from what they are at present before we can arrive at any accurate conclusion on the rate of mortality from different diseases. Such records, if accurately kept, could not fail to benefit the public; and it is to be hoped that Parliament will soon do something to remedy the defective state of our present mode of registering.*

* In concluding these remarks on the statistical history of consumption, I beg to express my obligations to my friend Mr. Fergus, to whom belongs the merit of collecting the numerous facts and constructing the tables contained in this chapter. They are the result of great research and founded on extensive calculations, and are highly creditable both to his ingenuity and industry.

CHAPTER IX.

THE history of tuberculous disease in animals is interesting to the physician, inasmuch as it affords a collateral illustration of the disease in man. Tubercles have been found in many orders of the Mammalia, carnivorous and herbivorous, in Birds, in Reptiles, and perhaps in Insects :—among the Mammalia, in the lion, dromedary, antelope, deer, horse, cow, sheep, goat, domestic pig, monkey, guinea-pig, hare, rabbit, squirrel, and porpoise : among birds, in the psittacus erythacus and some other macaws and parrots, in the flamingo, turkey, house-sparrow, and domestic fowl. Mr. Owen, Assistant Curator of the Museum of the Royal College of Surgeons, informs me that he has discovered tuberculous disease in the following animals which died in the Gardens of the Zoological Society,—felis caracal, *Persian lynx;* felis tigris, *tiger ;* paradoxurus typus, *paradoxure gennet;* viverra Rasse, *civet cat;* herpestes mungos, *Indian ichneumon;* nasua fusca, *brown coati mondi;* ursus Thibetanus, *Nepâl bear of the Himalaya Mountains;*

tapirus Americanus, *American tapir;* alces Americanus, *American elk;* simia satyrus, *ourang outang;* Macacus cynomolgus, *Macaque monkey;* M. radiatus, *bonnetted monkey;* M. Rhesus, *pig-tailed monkey;* cercopithecus sabæus, *green monkey;* papio maimon jun., *Mandrill baboon;* lemur nigrifrons, *black-fronted lemur;* lemur macauco, *ruffed macauco;* in an *Eskimaux dog,* and in the lungs of a large serpent (*Python tigris*).

The morbid appearances presented on examination of the animals enumerated bear a close analogy to those observed in man : the lungs, spleen, mucous membrane of the intestines, the liver, mesenteric, bronchial, and lymphatic glands, are the organs most frequently affected. We are, however, better acquainted with the morbid anatomy of monkeys, because, of all animals, that family is most subject to tuberculous disease; indeed, nearly all the monkeys in our menageries die tuberculous. Dr. Reynaud, of Paris, has made some interesting researches in this department of comparative pathology, and has published an excellent memoir on consumption in the monkeys at the Jardin des Plantes.* In fourteen of these animals he found the lungs containing tubercles, and in many cases they were almost entirely converted into tuberculous matter. In three monkeys the disease was confined to the lungs exclusively; in the others various organs were

* Archives de Médecine, t. xxv.

affected. The larynx was ulcerated in two cases; the bronchial glands were always more or less tuberculous, and in one instance they were so much enlarged as to obliterate the left bronchus and prevent respiration in the corresponding lung, which was much contracted. The spleen in six cases was much diseased, being enlarged and adherent to the peritoneum. The blood in the cells formed reddish clots, in the midst of which were tuberculous points. The tuberculous disease was found in various stages of softening, and sometimes there were caverns lined with a false membrane. In one case the tubercles in the lungs were isolated and crude, while in the spleen they were large and softened in the centre; showing that the spleen was the organ in which the tuberculous matter was first deposited.

As in the human species, so in animals the disease occurs at all ages. MM. Andral and Dupuy have even observed it in the fœtus of the sheep and rabbit.

My friend, Mr. Newport, a comparative anatomist of great promise, whose name is already favourably known by his researches into the minute anatomy of insects,* has favoured me with an account of what he believes to be tuberculous

---

* See his papers on the *Sphinx Ligustri*, in the Phil. Trans. 1833 and 1834.

deposits in that tribe. In the larva of the sphinx ligustri, or common privet moth, he met with a peculiar matter disseminated in small, irregular, aggregated masses, white, opaque, and of a cheesy consistence, over the whole internal surface of the insect, between layers of very delicate cellular tissue. These masses were most numerous among the muscles; on the exterior of the alimentary canal, particularly the stomach; on the secretory silk glands, in the biliary ducts, and on the nerves. In the carabus catenulatus, or ground-beetle, and in the staphylinus olens, both carnivorous feeders, he noticed similar deposits of more uniform and much smaller size in the cellular and pulmonary tissues: he also detected appearances similar to those observed in the sphinx ligustri, in the common cray-fish, the astacus fluviatilis of Leach. It is worthy of remark that the sphinx was fed upon stale leaves of the privet for some days previously to examination, the unusual wetness of the season having prevented a fresh supply.

While this chapter was passing through the press, I received the following additional observations from Mr. Newport, which I consider too important to be omitted; as they may be the means of calling the attention of others to this interesting subject.

" The concrete matter which I believe to be tuberculous is deposited chiefly between the layers of cellular tissue which surrounds the muscles and exists throughout the whole body of the insect: it is in the form of irregular, opaque, white masses, or granules. It sometimes occurs in the secretory organs, where it is much softer than when disseminated through other textures, and is of an opaque, white colour, very different from that of the natural secretions. When found in the salivary vessels and in the rudiments of the ovaries in the larva, it occurs in small patches, and in some specimens it has been observed in the salivary vessels only. The skin of the diseased insects (if in the state of larva) is generally slightly discoloured, dry, and shrivelled; and they are deficient in the plumpness of healthy individuals. In order to observe this substance, the insect should be placed in alcohol for a few days, during which time the matter becomes hardened, and is more readily distinguished from the fat and different textures.

" From the result of an experiment upon the larvæ of the *sphinx ligustri*, I am led to conclude that these depositions in insects may be produced almost at pleasure. About eighteen or twenty larvæ of this species, collected just after entering their last skin, were confined in a box closely covered and kept, uncleansed, in a room the temperature of which ranged from 65° to 80° Fahrenheit, and were supplied with food of deteriorated quality. By this means their growth and the period of their changing were retarded. In order to produce a sudden impression of cold upon them, they were repeatedly plunged into cold water.—The result was, that in the whole of them deposits were found, and generally in the secreting organs.

" Whatever may be the nature of this substance, it does not appear to be very common, in favourable seasons, in the larvæ of the sphinx while in their natural haunts. Upon examining many specimens, apparently quite healthy, soon after collecting them, I could find but few, perhaps scarcely one in ten, in which the disease was conspicuous.

" Since making these observations, I have discovered the disease in the common shrimp (*Cancer crangon:* Linn.) and in the scarce oil-beetle (*Meloë cicatricosus:* Linn.), both of which are vegetable feeders, the former feeding upon fuci and seaweed, and the latter upon the wild ranunculi, taraxicum, &c. The shrimps were collected from their natural haunts, and immediately placed in alcohol for preservation: upon examination some months afterwards, I found the disease more common in these instances than in any I have yet met with. The matter was disseminated in small granulated masses through the whole body, even within the substance of the nervous columns. In the meloë the masses existed upon the alimentary canal, hepatic vessels, and within the trachea, and there was one large mass, much softer than the

others, within the substance of the right supra-
œsophageal ganglion, or brain, occupying at least
one third of the ganglion itself."

Although the existence of tuberculous disease in
insects requires to be established by more numerous
observations than have as yet been made, still the
view which I take of the pathology of tuberculous
disease inclines me to believe that no class of
animals is exempt from it; I therefore have little
doubt that the application of causes analogous to
those which lead to it in the human species will also
induce it in any animal exposed to their influence.*

* All the milch cows in Paris, and no doubt elsewhere, become
tuberculous after a certain period of confinement. I have been
informed that for some time after the disease has commenced, the
quantity of milk obtained is greater than before, and that their
flesh is more esteemed by the unsuspecting epicure than that of
the healthy animal. A circumstance of the same kind is mentioned by Aristotle, who observed tubercles in the pig, the ox,
and the ass; in regard to strumous pigs, he says, that when the
disease *(grandines)* exists in a slight degree, the flesh is sweeter
(caro dulcior est). Historia Animalium, lib. viii. cap. 21.

CHAPTER X.

THE causes of tuberculous disease are referable to two distinct heads, the remote and the exciting,—those which induce the morbid state of the constitution,—tuberculous cachexia,—and those which determine the local deposition of tuberculous matter. The one class operates by modifying the whole system, the other by determining in a system so modified the particular morbid action of which tuberculous matter is the product. Until this distinction is fully understood, we shall make little progress in the prevention or treatment of tuberculous disease.

In a person little exposed to the exciting causes, the constitutional affection may long exist without any local disease; while their long-continued application may determine the local disease when the constitutional affection exists only in a slight degree. We have examples of the former in individuals among the wealthy classes, in whom tuberculous cachexia often prevails for a considerable time without the actual development of tubercles,

because they are little exposed to and even sedulously avoid the exciting causes : we meet with instances of the latter among the labouring classes,
such as those whose occupations compel them to
breathe for many hours a day an atmosphere
charged with fine particles of sand, metal, &c.,
by which pulmonary congestion and irritation are
induced. But too much importance has been attached to mechanical irritants in the production of
pulmonary consumption; they can only determine
the disease in those already constitutionally predisposed; and accordingly it will be found that the
most striking examples of consumption adduced as
the consequence of pulmonary irritation have occurred in individuals, who, together with the action
of mechanical irritants, were exposed to some of
the most powerful causes of tuberculous cachexia,
such as sedentary occupations carried on in a confined and deteriorated atmosphere, and abuse of
ardent spirits;—the causes of the constitutional
and local disease operating at the same time.

SECT. 1.—THE CAUSES OF TUBERCULOUS
CACHEXIA.

HEREDITARY ORIGIN.—That pulmonary consumption is an hereditary disease,—in other words,
that the tuberculous constitution is transmitted from

parent to child, is a fact not to be controverted; indeed,
I regard it as one of the best established points in
the etiology of the disease. A parent labouring
under tuberculous cachexia entails on his offspring
a disposition to the same affection, proportioned in
general to the degree of disease under which he
labours. Examples of this fact are constantly met
with in families of consumptive parents, where we
find the tuberculous constitution much more strongly
marked in general in the younger than in the elder
children. We even occasionally meet with families
in which the elder children are healthy, and the
younger are the subjects of tuberculous disease ;
the health of the parents having been deteriorated
during the increase of their family. There are,
no doubt, exceptions to this observation, depending
on circumstances beyond our cognizance, but frequently admitting of explanation in the state of the
parents' health. It has been questioned whether
the child is more disposed to the diseases of the
father or to those of the mother; and I believe the
majority of authors agree in favour of the former :
Professor Nasse of Bonn, however, in his excellent essay on tuberculous diseases, is of opinion
that the hereditary disposition is more frequently
derived from the mother. The point is very difficult of decision : there can be no doubt that the
child may inherit the constitution of either or both
parents ; on some occasions we see that of the

father, in others that of the mother, predominating in different children of the same family. It has also been remarked, and the observation appears to be correct, that the more a child resembles the parent in external lineaments, the more certainly will a disposition to the diseases of that parent prevail.

But a state of tuberculous cachexia is not the only morbid condition of the parent which entails the tuberculous predisposition on the children; there are several diseases which have this effect, the most important of which are a disordered state of the digestive organs, gout, cutaneous diseases, the injurious influence of mercury on the system, debility from disease, age, &c. ;—in short, a deteriorated state of health in the parent from any cause, to a degree sufficient to produce a state of cachexia, may give rise to the scrofulous constitution in the offspring.

However various may be the causes of the cachectic state of the parents, its effect is almost constantly manifested in the children by their evincing a predisposition to tuberculous disease. This is a very important circumstance in the history of consumption, and is highly deserving attentive consideration. In ascribing tuberculous disease in the offspring to an unhealthy state of the parent, I may appear disposed to generalize too much; but my opinion is not grounded upon superficial observation, or formed without mature reflection; and I am persuaded that when the subject is carefully investigated by others, my views will be found correct. We have frequent opportunities of noticing a strong disposition to scrofula in the children of those who enjoy what is usually termed good health, and in whose families no scrofulous taint can be traced; whereas, according to my observation, we never see the parents in an unhealthy state, whatever may be its nature, without finding, at the same time, that their children are strongly predisposed to tuberculous disease.

Of all diseases, I consider dyspepsia the most fertile source of cachexia of every form,—for this plain reason, that a healthy condition of the digestive organs, and a due performance of their functions are essential to the assimilation of food, and consequently to the supply of healthy nutriment. The adjusting powers of the system do much to correct a disordered condition of the different functions concerned in the process of assimilation and nutrition; but health cannot be long preserved when any one of these important functions is materially deranged.

A cachectic state may also originate in derangement of the various secretory and excretory functions, particularly that condition of them in which the effete matter is imperfectly carried off; and as this derangement very generally accompanies dyspepsia, it accelerates its deteriorating influence.

There are, doubtless, other circumstances in the state of the parents' health capable of giving rise to the strumous diathesis in their offspring, which are not so evident as those which I have noticed; but there can be little question of their influence, as we often see children presenting the characters of the strumous diathesis at the earliest age, while their parents are in the enjoyment of good health, and free from all appearances of tuberculous or other disease, constitutional or local. Remarkable examples of this kind have come under my observation, where whole families have fallen victims to tuberculous consumption, while the parents themselves enjoyed good health to an advanced age, and were unable to trace the existence of the disease in their families for generations back. An imperfect development or a feeble state of the organs of generation has been considered a cause of scrofula in the offspring;—any thing which interferes with the act of conception, or with the nourishment of the fœtus in utero,—such as a disordered state of the mother's health, depressing passions, a sedentary or unhealthy mode of life,—or whatever induces imperfect nutrition in the mother during pregnancy, may lead to such a result; and this may even explain why one child is predisposed to the disease, while the other children of the same family are exempt.

In the present state of our knowledge, it is not possible to determine the various circumstances in the health of the parent which may give rise to the scrofulous disposition in the child, much less to explain their mode of operation : I rather allude to them as subjects deserving the investigation of the general pathologist and practical physician. That tuberculous disease can generally be traced to an hereditary origin, that is, to a deteriorated state of health in the parent, will not be disputed by any medical observer who has attentively considered the subject; but there may be a difference of opinion as to the particular condition of the parent which induces the tuberculous constitution in the offspring, and also as to the degree in which this constitution may exist in the child at birth. Having stated my opinion respecting the former, I shall now give my views respecting the latter of these conditions.

1. We have seen, (p. 171,) that, although it is a rare occurrence, the child at birth may present tubercles in one or more of its organs.

2. The next degree of hereditary disease is that in which the infant is afflicted with tuberculous cachexia,—a state which requires very slight exciting causes to determine the deposition of tuberculous matter in some organ. The children of

consumptive parents are not unfrequently born in this state, and often die of tuberculous disease during the period of infancy.

3. Again, the child presents all the characters of the tuberculous or scrofulous constitution, and, without care, gradually lapses into a state of tuberculous cachexia, and dies of tuberculous disease. The greater number of scrofulous and consumptive cases which we meet with in childhood and youth are referable to this degree of hereditary predisposition.

4. In another class of cases, the child merely shows a predisposition to those functional derangements which generate the tuberculous constitution ; more especially to that form of dyspepsia (*strumous dyspepsia*) to which I have already referred, as capable of generating the tuberculous cachexia, and consequently of giving rise to every form of tuberculous or strumous disease. The cases of predisposition to consumption which come under this class are, according to my observation, the offspring of parents who have laboured under dyspepsia, gout, cutaneous, and other diseases not of a tuberculous nature. They constitute the most numerous and the most remediable of the degrees of hereditary disease; and yet their nature is generally the least understood.

I would beg to solicit the attention of the profession to the deteriorated health of the parent

as the origin of tuberculous disease : an acquaintance with the various derangements in the health
of the parent, and the mode and degree in which
these are manifested in the constitution of their
offspring, is requisite to enable us to obviate them,
and thereby to correct the hereditary predisposition.

An opinion is entertained that one generation
sometimes escapes hereditary tuberculous disease,
while the immediately preceding and succeeding
generations are the subjects of it. This is not a
very common occurrence, and, when properly investigated, would, I have no doubt, admit of a
satisfactory explanation, without supposing that
the disease lay dormant in one generation to manifest itself in the next.

SECT. II.—THE CAUSES OF TUBERCULOUS CA-CHEXIA IN INDIVIDUALS NOT HEREDITARILY PREDISPOSED.

Having, in the preceding section, taken a view
of the hereditary causes of tuberculous disease, I
shall now notice the causes of the disease in persons
exempt from hereditary predisposition.

In childhood, the earlier the causes of tuberculous cachexia are applied, the more speedily will it
be induced. If, for example, an infant, born in
perfect health and of the healthiest parents, be

insufficiently or injudiciously fed, that is, be nursed
by a woman whose milk is inadequate in quantity
or quality to afford proper nourishment; (it may
be too rich and too exciting, or it may not be sufficiently nutritious;)—or if the child be fed on other
food ill-suited to the state of the digestive organs,
or be confined to rooms in which free ventilation
and cleanliness are neglected, a few months will
often suffice to induce tuberculous cachexia. The
countenance will become pale, the flesh soft, the
limbs emaciated, the abdomen tumid, and the
evacuations fetid and unnatural. The external
lymphatic glands, especially those of the neck, will
enlarge, and the child will speedily fall a victim
to tuberculous disease, while its brothers and sisters,
who have been properly suckled and reared with
care, attain a healthy maturity. If this is the case
in a strong infant, the offspring of healthy parents,
and perfectly healthy at its birth, how much more
certainly and rapidly will the same effects be produced in the feeble infant, of unhealthy parents,
or, still more, of parents absolutely scrofulous?
Again, take a child of three or four years of age,
in perfect health, having been born without any
hereditary predisposition to disease, well nursed,
and hitherto properly nourished,—let it be fed upon
coarse innutritious food, and confined in close ill-
ventilated apartments, where neither the heat nor
light of the sun has free admission, and we shall

soon see the healthy blooming child changed into a pale, sickly, leucophlegmatic object.* During the whole period of youth the same condition may be induced, although, as we advance in life, a longer time is requisite to effect such constitutional deterioration. But up to the period of the full development of the system, until the body has ceased to increase in stature,—has reached maturity and acquired the stability of the adult, tuberculous cachexia may be readily induced. After maturity the powers of the system in resisting the causes of disease are greater than at an earlier age; still we see the same results produced by similar causes,— the constitutional affection being the same, although it is induced more slowly and manifests itself in a different manner, according to the age and peculiar constitution of the individual.

The principal causes which induce tuberculous disease may be arranged under the heads of improper diet, impure air, deficient exercise, imperfect

---

* The same is observed in the lower animals. It is well known that cows confined in close stables in towns become tuberculous, and would die consumptive if not sold to the butcher in the commencement of the disease; and that rabbits may be rendered tuberculous in the course of a few weeks, by confining them in a close humid place, and feeding them on innutritious food; and they are often as speedily cured by removing them to a well-aired, dry situation, and giving them nutritious food.

clothing, inattention to cleanliness, abuse of spirituous liquors, and affections of the mind.

IMPROPER DIET.—The most powerful are those
causes which interfere with the due nutrition of the
body. An imperfect supply of food, or food of an
innutritious quality, forms a very efficient cause,
although we have rarely an opportunity of observing
the effects of this alone; because when the means
of procuring proper nourishment are wanting, other
causes are generally in action at the same time,
such as residence in ill-ventilated and dark apartments, exposure to cold from imperfect clothing,
&c.; all of which are often combined, and hence
more speedily effect the deterioration of the health.
But proper food, when taken in excess, or when of
too exciting a quality, may also induce tuberculous
cachexia in youth,—a circumstance which is not
sufficiently attended to,—I may say not generally
understood, even by medical men; nevertheless I
hold it to be a frequent cause of scrofula. Imperfect digestion and excitement of the digestive
organs in the one case, and inadequate supply of
nourishment in the other, lead ultimately to a
similar state of disease:—the form and general
character which it assumes may differ, but in both
cases the result may be the same. The adaptation
of the food, in quality and quantity, to the age of
the individual, as well as to the powers of the digestive organs, is too little considered, and the evil

consequences of this neglect are often evinced in the children of the wealthy classes, who are frequently allowed an unrestricted use of the most exciting kinds of animal food, than which there cannot be a greater error. By a too-stimulating diet at this early age the digestive organs become over-excited; the biliary and other secretions connected with digestion are diminished; congestion of the abdominal circulation ensues; and the skin, sympathising with the irritation of the internal surfaces, becomes dry and harsh, and cutaneous eruptions, or copious perspiration, are common consequences. The ultimate effect is often tuberculous disease, which is generally attributed to imperfect nourishment; and on this erroneous view steel and other tonics and stimulants are often prescribed, by which the evil is increased.

IMPURE AIR.—Next to improper or deficient diet, I would rank an imperfect supply of pure air. The assimilation of the chyle, or nutritious element of our food, is completed during its circulation through the lungs, and by being brought into contact with the atmospheric air in the process of respiration. It is, therefore, quite evident, that when respiration is imperfectly performed, from a defective action of the respiratory organs,—the consequence of disease, of a sedentary life, or of unnatural position of the body,—or from an imperfect supply of pure air, perfect assimilation cannot be effected.

In the confined districts of large and populous cities, where neither pure air nor sufficient light can enter in consequence of the obscure and over-shaded sites of the buildings, the food of the inhabitants cannot be assimilated even though the supply be unexceptionable. A sensible writer on scrofulous diseases considers impure air as their only real cause; other causes may assist, but this he considers essential to their production.*

Although I admit the powerful influence of impure air in the production of scrofula, I cannot entirely coincide with M. Baudelocque. I feel satisfied that the other causes which have been mentioned are capable of inducing scrofula, while the patient is breathing a very pure air. The disease not unfrequently affects the inhabitants of elevated and dry countries, where the atmosphere is pure, and where the people, being occupied in

---

* " Telle est la véritable cause, la seule cause, peut-être, de la maladie scrophuleuse·········partout où il y a des scrophu-leux cette cause existe, que partout où elle existe, il y a des scrophuleux, et que là où elle manque la maladie scrophuleuse n'est pas connue." *Etudes sur les Causes, la Nature, et le Traitement de la Maladie Scrophuleuse, par A. C. Baude-locque, Docteur et Agrégé de la Faculté de Médecine de Paris, Médecin de l'Hôpital des Enfans, &c. &c.* Paris, 1834.

grazing sheep and cattle, are so much in the open air, and the purest air also, during the day, that the confined atmosphere of their close hovels can scarcely be considered the chief cause. Other and more evident causes exist in the coarse and innutritious vegetable food which forms almost their only sustenance, in their scanty clothing and their exposure to the inclemency of the weather. But there can be no doubt that the habitual respiration of the air of confined and gloomy alleys in large towns, as well as of that of many manufactories, of workhouses, and schools, and of our nurseries and very sitting-rooms, is a powerful means of augmenting the hereditary predisposition to scrofula, and of inducing such a disposition *de novo*. Almost all the children reared in the workhouses of this country and in similar establishments abroad become scrofulous,—more, I believe, from the impure atmosphere which they breathe, and the want of sufficient exercise, than from defective nourishment.

Were I to select two circumstances which influence the health, especially during the growth of the body, more than any others, and concerning which the public generally, at present most ignorant of them, ought to be well informed, they would be the proper adaptation of food to difference of age and constitution, and the constant supply of pure air for respiration.

DEFICIENT EXERCISE.—Deficient exercise ranks

next as a cause of tuberculous disease. If a due supply of proper food and pure air are necessary to nutrition, bodily exercise is scarcely less so to ensure the proper growth and development of the body. The amount of exercise necessary to produce this effect, and to maintain a healthy state of the system, will vary according to the age and the constitution of the individual; but without exercise we have abundant proof that there cannot be sound health, more particularly in early life.

EXCESSIVE LABOUR.—While a certain quantity of exercise is necessary to the maintenance of health, excessive labour, particularly in early age, may be ranked as a cause of disease. It exhausts and debilitates, and in youth checks the full growth and development of the body. When labour is carried on in confined apartments, its injurious effects are more decided and more rapid.

IMPERFECT CLOTHING. — Proper clothing is essential to the preservation of health in civilized life. An imperfectly protected state of the body in the cold season, especially when the individual is engaged in a sedentary occupation, and has not exercise sufficient to sustain the circulation of the fluids, is most injurious, particularly to young persons, in whom a vigorous circulation through the extreme parts of the body is essential in order to promote its growth and development, to secure the due performance of the cutaneous functions, and to prevent sanguineous congestion of the internal organs. These objects cannot be effected without exercise and warm clothing. While on this point, although the subject has become trite, I cannot abstain from noticing the pernicious effects of the modern system of female dress. Since the free expansion of the chest,—in other words, the unimpeded action of the organs of respiration,—is essential to health, the employment of tight stays and other forms of dress which interfere with these natural actions must be injurious, and cannot, therefore, be too strongly censured.*

WANT OF CLEANLINESS.—Inattention to cleanliness is another common cause of disease, and although it may be less powerful than those just mentioned, still it has its influence. Without cleanliness it is obvious that the cutaneous functions cannot be properly performed: the effects of a deranged state of these functions in the production of tuberculous disease have been already explained.

ABUSE OF SPIRITUOUS LIQUORS.—Among the causes of tuberculous cachexia, a free indulgence in ardent spirits holds an important place. While this pernicious habit is one of the most powerful means of debasing the morals of the people and of extinguishing the best feelings of human nature,

---

* I beg to refer to the excellent article on PHYSICAL EDUCATION in the *Cyclopædia of Practical Medicine*, by Dr. Barlow, for some very judicious observations on this subject.

it is no less effective in destroying the physical
constitution. There is good reason to believe that
the abuse of spirituous liquors among the lower
classes in this country is productive of consumptive
and other tuberculous diseases to an extent far
beyond what is usually imagined. The blanched
cadaverous aspect of the spirit-drinker bespeaks
the condition of his internal organs. The tale of
his moral and physical degradation is indelibly
written on his countenance. The evil unfortunately
does not rest with him: by destroying his own
health, he entails on his unhappy offspring the
disposition to tuberculous disease.

MENTAL CAUSES.—Intense application to study
is a powerful cause of tuberculous diseases. This
operates in several ways: it necessarily implies
sedentary habits, and, consequently, liability to all
the evils which arise from them, such as imperfect
digestion, constipated bowels, &c. The sensorial
power, moreover, is so much exhausted as to
weaken the nervous system, and to deprive the
various organs, the functions of which are essential
to health, of their due proportions of nervous
influence. Mental depression also holds a very
conspicuous place among those circumstances which
diminish the powers of the system generally, and
it often proves one of the most effectual determining causes of consumption. Disappointment of
long-cherished hopes, slighted affections, loss of

dear relations, and reverse of fortune, often exert a powerful influence on persons predisposed to consumption, more particularly in the female sex.

Various other causes of consumptive diseases have been noticed by authors. Hard water, that is, water holding an unusual quantity of calcareous matter in solution, has been considered as such, and the evidences adduced in proof of this appear to me sufficient to show that it has an influence in the production of scrofula. The effects of the water at Rheims, related in the Memoirs of the Royal Society of Medicine at Paris, have often been adduced as a striking example.* Heberden† and Cullen have both noticed the influence of this cause;‡ and we may refer the reader to the various works of Dr. Lambe, who has gone into minute details on this subject. It may be difficult to explain how hard water produces such an effect; but the fact should be sufficient to guide us in the selection of a residence for children, more especially for those predisposed to tuberculous disease, or to the disordered state of the digestive organs which engenders it.

Mercury, when used so as to affect the system, has been very generally considered capable of in-

* Mém. de Soc. Royale de Méd. vol. ii. p. 280.
† Commentaries, p. 362.
‡ Materia Medica, vol. i. p. 406.

ducing tuberculous disease. I am inclined to
believe this, and therefore consider that in persons
of a delicate or strumous constitution its use requires the greatest caution and circumspection.

There are, no doubt, various other circumstances
which debilitate the system generally and predispose to consumption;—among these may be
mentioned the excesses of youth, which especially
debilitate the nervous system, and which, although
they occasionally induce an atrophy of a peculiar
character, much more frequently induce that general
depression of the vital powers which favours the
production of tuberculous disease.

Contagion.—The contagious nature of consumption has been believed by some authors of high
authority, at the head of whom may be placed
Morgagni, and altogether disbelieved by others.
In the south of Europe the general opinion is in
favour of contagion, in the north of Europe against
it. As the subject scarcely admits of being confirmed or refuted, and as every medical man in this
country has too frequent opportunities of making
his own observations and forming his own judgment
upon it, it would be profitless to adduce authorities
or detail opinions. The view which I take of tuberculous cachexia, without which, in my opinion,
tuberculous disease of the lungs cannot occur, leads
me entirely to disbelieve that consumption can be
communicated by contagion. But I consider the
practice of sleeping in the same bed, or even in

the same room with a patient in the advanced stage
of consumption, highly objectionable, because the
rooms of the consumptive are rendered peculiarly
injurious to health by the nature of the disease,
and the confined atmosphere and high temperature
in which they are too often kept.

Seeing that the causes which produce tuberculous
cachexia are so numerous, we should be extremely
cautious in estimating their individual influence,
and in attributing to any of them specific powers.
Whenever their combined effect is such as to
depress the vital energy, and lower the power of
assimilation beyond a certain degree, the tuberculous diathesis will be induced : whenever, on
the contrary, the nutritive functions are vigorously
carried on, this disposition will not manifest itself,
however strongly it may be favoured by the separate
action of any one of the causes, in the degree in
which it is usually applied.

SECT. III.—CAUSES DETERMINING TUBERCULOUS

DISEASE OF THE LUNGS.

The chief causes that come under this head are
certain diseases which may be divided into two
classes,—those which act immediately on the lungs,
and those which act partly on the lungs, and partly
on the general system.

The pulmonary diseases, of which tubercles are considered as the result, are inflammation of the bronchial membrane and of the substance of the lungs, and hemorrhage.

BRONCHITIS.—Irritation and inflammation of the mucous membrane of the larynx, trachea, and bronchi, is considered a frequent cause of consumption: certain it is that no affection so commonly appears to precede it as bronchial irritation. This circumstance may be accounted for in two ways: first, the pulmonary mucous membrane of tuberculous subjects is very susceptible of the impressions of causes which produce congestion and irritation, such as vicissitudes in the temperature and humidity of the atmosphere, or mechanical irritants conveyed into the air-passages during respiration;—and, secondly, tubercles often prove a source of bronchial irritation long before their presence is indicated by other symptoms. But I admit that repeated attacks of bronchial inflammation, or the long continued application of mechanical irritants to the membrane of the bronchi, may prove the exciting cause of consumption, when the constitutional predisposition exists.

Different portions of the mucous membrane of the air-passages may be the primary seat of irritation. In some persons the larynx is first affected, the irritation gradually extending to the trachea and bronchi. In this case the patient is subject to frequent attacks of laryngeal irritation, which are usually excited by exposure to a cold humid atmosphere. There is a sensation of uneasiness in the larynx, shortly followed by an increased secretion of mucus, with frequent hawking to remove it; generally, also, there is more or less hoarseness, and some degree of cough. In other cases the person has repeated attacks of inflammation of the internal fauces, from whence the disease seems to extend to the larynx. At length, an attack, more obstinate than the others, remains, and is soon accompanied by a cough; or if cough existed previously, it increases in severity; and the uneasy sensations, at first confined to the larynx, are now felt under the upper part of the sternum, and soon extend over the chest. The cough gradually becomes deeper and more troublesome, calling into action all the muscles of respiration, and medicine does little more than palliate it. A patient may continue in this state for a considerable time without fever or any alarming symptom; but his appearance generally indicates that there is more than bronchial disease.

Such a patient is commonly said to have an " affection of the trachea," although in truth the tracheal portion of the mucous membrane when affected produces little irritation; for extensive ulceration is frequently found in this part when there were no signs of its presence during life.

In another class of cases (and these are the most
numerous) the morbid state of the mucous membrane commences in, and is chiefly confined to the
bronchi ; the larynx and trachea appearing to be
little affected. The patient is liable to pulmonary
catarrh on the slightest exposure to cold ; during
the whole winter and spring attack succeeds attack,
with scarcely any cessation of cough. This state
often continues for many years in persons, even in
those of a tuberculous constitution, without terminating in consumption, and has been termed tuberculous bronchitis. The subjects of these chronic
bronchial affections, when occurring in early life,
are generally persons of great delicacy of constitution. Their cases are extremely embarrassing, and
without the aid of the physical signs of pulmonary
disease, the medical attendant will often remain
long ignorant of the nature of the disease.

With care such patients may be preserved for
many years ; but sooner or later the catarrhal affection becomes permanent, the respiration is more
oppressed, the pulse is habitually frequent, and
the emaciation, which had varied according to the
severity or duration of the catarrhal attacks, and
the length of the intervening cessation, now remains or progressively increases. The aspect of the
patient is also much changed, and the symptoms
collectively announce the establishment of tuberculous disease in the lungs.

These cases afford the strongest evidence of the influence of bronchial irritation in producing consumption ; and I have no doubt that when the least predisposition to tuberculous disease exists, long-continued irritation of the bronchial membrane leads to the deposition of tuberculous matter in the extreme branches of the bronchi and the air-cells. But, as M. Andral observes, " what ought never to be lost sight of is this, that in order that inflammation of the mucous membranes of the air-passages shall be followed by the production of pulmonary tubercles, it is necessary to admit a predisposition. This being admitted, we can easily conceive how in one individual very slight bronchitis is sufficient to produce tubercles, whilst others do not become phthisical from the most severe and long-continued pulmonary catarrh."*

The bronchial affections just noticed are met with in all conditions of life, and mostly result from exposure to a cold and humid atmosphere, or the alternation of this with the air of heated rooms. Breathing an atmosphere loaded with particles of matter which mechanically irritate and excite permanent disease of the bronchial membrane, has been already noticed as another fruitful source of bronchial irritation.

PNEUMONIA.—Inflammation of the pulmonary

* Clinique Médicale, t. ii. p. 32.

tissue is considered a frequent, and, by some
authors, the chief cause of consumption. So generally, indeed, has this opinion prevailed, and so
injurious has it proved, and continues to prove, to
the progress of our knowledge, and, consequently,
to the rational treatment of tuberculous consumption, that I consider it of the greatest importance
to show its fallacy. With this view I willingly
avail myself of the opinion of Dr. Carswell, than
whom no pathologist has investigated the subject
with more care, or with a mind more perfectly un-
influenced by any theoretical bias. After pointing
out the necessity of making a distinction between
the localization of disease in an organ, and the
morbid condition of the economy in which such
disease originates and from which it derives its
peculiar character, he proceeds :—" The presence
of tuberculous matter constitutes the material element of the disease now under consideration, and
like every other morbid product of the same class,
has its peculiar and distinctive characters. It is in
consequence of the tuberculous matter presenting
these peculiar characters, that we consider it to be
a disease *sui generis ;* and it is also in consequence
of this matter being formed in particular organs,
as it were indifferently (at least as regards the
rapidity and extent of its formation), under every
variety of morbid agency to which these organs
may have been subjected, that we cannot admit its

formation to be the necessary consequence of any of those local causes to which it has been ascribed. Were we to examine these causes in detail, we should find that there is no necessary connection between any one of them and the formation of tuberculous matter. The most obvious of these causes, and that to which by far the greatest importance has been attached, is inflammation, or certain real or imaginary modifications of it. Now it is well known to every practical pathologist whose mind is not biassed by preconceived theory, that inflammation, whatever may have been the tissue or organ affected with it, is not necessarily followed by the formation of tuberculous matter or any other product of a similar kind, inasmuch as in such cases we often meet with no trace of this particular product in the affected organ after death; and, on the contrary, the formation of tuberculous matter is found to take place in organs, the functions of which were never observed to have been deranged, and in which, after death, none of those lesions could be detected which are known to follow inflammation. Under such circumstances it would be absurd to ascribe the origin of tuberculous matter to inflammation—an effect and its cause are always inseparable under conditions of a similar kind. Applying this law to the solution of the question before us, we arrive at a fact which of itself is sufficient to overthrow every argument which has been brought forward in support of the local origin of tuberculous disease, and which supersedes the necessity of those researches which have been made to prove or disprove such a theory, by determining the relative frequency and order of succession of local lesion and functional derangement, observed in the affected organ, viz. *that the products of inflammation are always the same under conditions of a similar kind.* These products are *coagulable lymph* or *pus ;* and that inflammation has always a tendency towards the formation of one or both of these products, is proved by the infinitely more frequent occurrence of these than of any other morbid product, consequent on this physiological change. We are therefore entitled to conclude that pus and coagulable lymph are the *natural products* of inflammation, and that, were the conditions under which this pathological state takes place always the same, its products would be so also. Hence it follows that when other products than these make their appearance in inflammation, the legitimate conclusion is, that some other morbid condition besides inflammation is present, and to this morbid condition alone must be owing the essential and distinctive characters of such products."*

It is almost unnecessary to add, that my views are perfectly in accordance with those of Dr. Cars-

---

* Op. citat.

well. Although I believe that tuberculous matter
is never a product of inflammation in a healthy
person, I am of opinion that inflammation may and
often does prove a determining cause in a tuberculous
constitution; and on this account the utmost care
should be taken to prevent its occurrence in such
subjects, and to remove it when it has taken place.
Pneumonic inflammation is one of the worst evils
that can befal a patient already labouring under
tuberculous disease of the lungs, as it never fails to
increase the mischief, and frequently converts that
which was latent, and might have long remained
so, into active disease. It promotes the softening of the tubercles, and renders the pulmonary
tissue at once incapable of the functions of respiration, and a fit nidus for the further deposition of
tuberculous matter. Indeed, I shall not err far, I
believe, in stating, that in proportion to the extent
of pneumonic inflammation, will be in general the
rapidity of consumption. It is chiefly in those
persons who, without suffering from extreme debility, are little liable to inflammation, that we observe consumption protracted to a great length,—the
tuberculous disease reaching a considerable extent
without producing much febrile disturbance.

HEMOPTYSIS.—I have already remarked, that
pathologists differ in their opinions respecting the
influence of hemoptysis, some regarding pulmonary
hemorrhage as the consequence, others the cause, of

tubercles. M. Andral believes hemoptysis to be at
once a proof and consequence of pulmonary congestion, a state which he considers necessary to
the formation of tubercles; and having also on
several occasions found, both in man and in the
horse, tubercles deposited in a coagulum of blood
in the lungs, he concludes that in this way the
effusion of blood may become an exciting cause.

If we attend to the history of the cases in which
hemoptysis occurs, there will generally be sufficient
evidence to show that it is a consequence of tubercles in the lungs, or at least that it occurs subsequently to their formation ; although it may originate in simple pulmonary congestion. It is to be
regretted that in the accounts of this and other
diseases adduced as causes of consumption, the
patient's previous health and the diseases of his
family are not stated. The cases of French authors,
which, in other respects, are detailed with praise-
worthy care and minuteness, are often defective on
this point. This is, indeed, a kind of information
which is not sufficiently appreciated, and I have
had constantly to lament the want of it in my examination of works on the subject of this treatise.
From omitting to inquire into the previous health
of consumptive patients, the constitutional origin
of the disease has been overlooked, or undervalued,
and undue importance attached to diseases of the
lungs as causes.

I now proceed to notice various diseases affecting the general system, which have been considered capable of giving rise to phthisis.

FEVER.—Fevers, both continued and intermittent, are not infrequently followed so closely by consumption as to make them appear exciting causes. Portal gives a chapter on a form of consumption induced by such fevers ; yet the cases which he has adduced, chiefly from Lieutaud, are not cases of simple fever, but of fever complicated with inflammation of the lungs and pleura, followed by tuberculous disease. Independently, however, of such complications, it often happens that symptoms of consumption are observed for the first time towards the termination of, or during the convalescence from, fever.

Fever occurring in a person of tuberculous constitution may prove the exciting cause of tuberculous deposits in the lungs, from the irritation and congestion to which these organs are exposed in such a state of the system. In this case, when the fever goes through its usual course favourably, the febrile symptoms abate, the tongue may become moist and clean, the skin soft, and the various secretions natural ; but there is a slight return of fever towards evening, and the pulse is frequent at all times : still the patient seems on the verge of convalescence, and the medical attendant expects to find the pulse slower at each visit, and generally predicts speedy recovery. He is, however, disappointed: the frequency of the pulse increases; the evening accessions become more marked; there is a circumscribed flush on the cheek different from the general flush of fever, and there are occasional chills: the slight cough which attended the fever increases; perspirations occur towards morning; and the breathing is observed to be more rapid than during the height of the fever. The real state of things now becomes evident. The original fever has ceased, but in place of terminating in recovery, as would have been the result in a healthy subject, it is immediately succeeded by, or rather lapses into, hectic fever. The patient, already greatly reduced, becomes an easy victim to tuberculous disease of the lungs, and generally sinks rapidly under it.

The rapid progress of consumption, occurring after fever, very often depends upon the previous existence of tuberculous disease of the lungs in a latent state. The irritation of the mucous membranes of the lungs and digestive organs, which generally accompanies fevers, favours the increase of the tuberculous disease, and the state of convalescence renders the person extremely susceptible of the exciting causes of pulmonary congestion.

There are other cases in which the fever appears connected with the occurrence of phthisis, inasmuch as the patient never after regains his strength, although many months may elapse before he shows decided indications of tuberculous disease. In this case the fever probably acts more as a remote or predisposing than as an exciting cause of the disease.

There remains to be noticed a febrile affection which is peculiar to childhood, at least in its more acute form, and which is fraught with the utmost danger, as it proves a frequent exciting cause of tuberculous disease : I allude to what is commonly denominated *infantile remittent fever.* This, if neglected or improperly treated, often induces fatal cerebral disease ; but it more frequently assumes a chronic form, and being essentially seated in the digestive organs, speedily leads to a derangement of the digestive function and the various secretions connected with it, and moreover renders the child extremely liable to acute attacks of gastric and bronchial irritation, from slight errors in diet, exposure to cold, &c. This affection is considered by Hufeland to be so intimately connected with tuberculous disease, that he regards it as a precursor of the scrofulous diathesis, or a sign of its presence, and proposes to name it scrofulous fever. According to his observation, it is most frequent within the two first years of life.*

Eruptive fevers, particularly rubeola, scarla-

* Traité de la Maladie Scrophuleuse, p. 92.

tina, and variola, occurring in persons of a tuberculous constitution, are attended with still greater
danger than continued fever.

RUBEOLA.—Bronchial disease, often of a very
severe character, forms an essential part of measles,
so that we have bronchial irritation superadded to
the fever. In early life measles are known to prove
a frequent exciting cause of tuberculous disease,
and in persons constitutionally predisposed to consumption, the greatest attention should be paid to
the state of convalescence from them, for it is
during this period that the danger of pulmonary
disease is most imminent, and accordingly consumption in many cases is not unjustly attributed
to the effects of measles.

SCARLATINA.—Although attended with less bronchial irritation, scarlatina is still a very dangerous
disease to young persons disposed to, or labouring
under, the tuberculous diathesis. During convalescence from scarlatina there is a peculiar disposition to inflammation, and pleurisy and pneumonia
are easily induced by slight exposure to cold, fatigue,
and similar causes, for some time after the eruption
has ceased; the lymphatic system is also peculiarly
liable to disease. The rapidity of consumption
after scarlatina, which was noticed by Morton, is,
I believe, chiefly owing to the inflammation of the
pleura or lungs being superadded to the tuberculous
disease previously existing. I repeat that it is

during the convalescence from these diseases that the greatest danger is to be apprehended; the most sedulous care, therefore, should be taken during that period to guard against exposure to cold and other exciting causes of pulmonary congestion and irritation.

VARIOLA.—Small-pox is generally accompanied with much bronchial irritation, and proves a very fatal disease in the strumous habit; but fortunately we have few opportunities of witnessing the evil consequences of it at present.

Several other diseases have been considered causes of phthisis, such as *rheumatism, syphilis, psora,* &c.; but the observations upon which this opinion rests do not appear to have been made with sufficient accuracy to merit much attention.

CHAPTER XI.

PATHOLOGY OF CONSUMPTION AND TUBERCULOUS
DISEASES IN GENERAL.

IN a certain condition of the system, which I have
endeavoured to describe under the title of tuberculous cachexia, a peculiar matter is poured out by
the extreme vessels, and is deposited in the various
tissues and organs of the body. This matter, constituting one of the modes in which the morbid
modification of the general system manifests itself,
observes laws of formation, and presents physical
characters, by which, however it may be affected in
form and appearance by the structure or functions of
different organs, it can generally be recognised.

The disease, of which this matter constitutes the
distinctive anatomical character, has received different names according to its development in particular organs and tissues. In the external glands
and in the bones, it is commonly called scrofula ;
in the lungs, phthisis ; and in the glands of the
mesentery, tabes, &c. By the ancients, the identity of these affections was only suspected, from the
similarity of the general symptoms ; but by modern

pathologists it has been established on the clear evidence of morbid anatomy ;—an increased attention to which science, and a closer study of the causes of tuberculous disease, have led to more accurate opinions and more comprehensive views regarding it.

From the rounded form which this matter assumes in certain situations, it received the inappropriate name of *tubercle;* a term still applied to it by modern pathologists, although designating an appearance occasionally assumed by other morbid products, and not constant in this, but depending chiefly, as has been already stated, on the structure of the parts in which it is deposited.

This matter, however denominated, is now generally considered by the best pathologists as a morbid unorganizable product, having for its remote or predisposing cause a cachectic state of the general system, and for its immediate production some anormal action of the vessels of the part in which it is deposited, but with the nature of which action we are not acquainted. No constitution, no temperament, age, sex, or race, as we have already seen, is entirely exempt from the liability to this disease, although the disposition to it is strongest in that condition of the body called lymphatic, in the age of infancy, in the female sex, and in the negro race.

In whatever light we may regard tuberculous

cachexia, we shall find that its phenomena are
explicable only by admitting that it depends on a
general modification of the whole animal economy ;
and that the notion of its being the morbid degeneration of any organ or tissue, or of any particular
system, or the morbid modification of any single
fluid, is founded on limited views of its nature and
laws. The deposition of tuberculous matter in any
of the tissues or organs of the body is the result of
previous changes in the general system, cognizable,
as I have endeavoured to show (Chap. I.), by the
physical condition of the patient, — a condition
quite distinct from mere debility, and therefore in-
explicable on the idea of a difference of force or
tone of the system ; and which, though very generally accompanied with a feeble organisation, is not
inconsistent with too great development and inordinate action of particular parts, and even with
considerable physical power of the system.

The universality of the peculiar condition of the
system just referred to, necessarily modifies the
structure of every part, the nature of every fluid,
and the qualities of every secretion. The osseous
system is more spongy ; the muscular is flaccid and
imperfectly developed ; the cellular tissue is singu-
larly lax ; the vascular system is weak and irregular
in its action, and is subject to local congestions
from the slightest causes : the skin is generally thin
and soft, or thick, coarse, and dry, and is affected

by various diseases, apparently arising from the morbid condition of its function of secretion, which, in tuberculous subjects, is always more or less deranged. The mucous system is peculiarly susceptible of disease ; and, on the application of the slightest causes of irritation or congestion, matter, differing more or less from the healthy secretion, is poured forth in large quantities from the surfaces of the mucous membranes. The blood is serous, and deficient in fibrine and colouring matter.* The lymphatic system, being more intimately concerned in the function of nutrition, is more peculiarly affected ; and hence it has been by many considered as the original seat of the disease.

These morbid conditions of both fluids and solids are examples and proofs of a defective organisation. In the healthy state of the nutritive function each part separates the materials proper for its nutrition, and converts them into its own particular tissue or structure; and the various secreting organs secrete their peculiar fluids,—some to be applied to the purposes of the animal economy, others to serve as vehicles for eliminating effete and useless matter from the system. It is necessary to the maintenance of health that both these functions,—the nutritive and excretory;—should be performed in a certain ratio:

* Andral, Anat. Path. Trans. vol. 1. p. 535.

and thus it may happen that imperfect assimilation on the one hand, or defective secretion and elimination on the other, shall give rise to such a disordered state of the constitution as may ultimately terminate in tuberculous cachexia.

This comprehensive view of the nature and causes of tuberculous cachexia, and of its influence on the secretions and on the products of diseased action, leads to the conclusion that tuberculous deposits are always at first fluid, and that the concrete form, in which they are commonly found, arises simply from the absorption of the more fluid part, and is in many situations dependent chiefly on compression, as is shown, (p. 122); and I have no difficulty in conceiving that the matter formed in certain cutaneous eruptions, and that thrown off from the free surfaces of mucous membranes, would have assumed all the characters of crude tubercle, had it been confined in the parenchyma of organs, or the extreme bronchial ramifications, &c.

I shall here give Dr. Todd's theory of the production of tubercles, which most satisfactorily deduces their deposition from a defective function of nutrition, and is in accordance with all the phenomena of the morbid condition of body by which they are induced. From his experiments on the reproduction of the amputated extremities of the aquatic salamander, Dr. Todd was led to the conclusion that nutrition consists of two distinct processes,—the secretion and deposition of a fluid matrix, the same as coagulable lymph, and the organization of this lymph, or its conversion into organised tissue. Though not to be distinctly as-certained in the ordinary process of nutrition, Dr. Todd thinks that, from the analogy of the growth and organization of the chick in ovo, of the fœtus, of the union of divided, and the nutrition of lost parts, these two processes always co-operate in the performance of the function of nutrition. Now if from any cause or combination of causes, a gene-ral morbid condition of the system shall arise, from which the constitution of the blood—the fountain from which this matrix is secreted—or the action of the vessels—the power by which it is secreted—should be imperfect, it is easy to understand how this nutritive matrix, either from deficient vitality or some other condition, may be formed of a nature below the standard of organization, and how in this state the nutritive molecules may, instead of tissue, be converted into tubercles.—This is the general outline of Dr. Todd's theory of the forma-tion of tubercles : for a fuller account of it I must refer to my work on Climate.*

The foregoing observations, with some slight ex-ceptions, are to be regarded rather as a detail of

---

* Influence of Climate, p. 311.

the more constant phenomena which accompany
the development and progress of tuberculous
disease, than as an exposition of its real pathology.
If, in the following remarks, I should deviate from
the strict path of demonstrable fact, I shall still be
borne out, I believe, by observation and by the
results of practical experience; but I am even
willing to incur the imputation of yielding a little
to theory rather than leave unsaid that which I am
disposed to think may be of practical value to
some of my readers.

It is reasonable to believe that the remote causes
of consumption and of tuberculous disease in general, however various their mode of operation may
appear, act by inducing some peculiar or determinate derangement of the system,—some positive
pathological condition or conditions, which, being
constantly present wherever tuberculous disease is
found, may be regarded as necessary to its production.   Although I readily admit that we cannot fix
on any pathological condition, the presence of
which is absolutely necessary to the production of
tuberculous cachexia, there is one so very generally
present as in a practical point of view to demand
our especial attention.   I allude to a state of congestion of the venous system of the abdomen,
which has been termed abdominal plethora.

In the present defective state of our knowledge
of the laws which regulate the animal economy,

we can neither trace the various functional disorders which lead to abdominal congestion, nor understand the processes which connect it with tuberculous cachexia. But although we cannot perceive every link of the chain, we have, I am persuaded, a good notion of the chain itself. It is not, I think, difficult to understand how abdominal plethora, by impeding the functions of the nutritive organs and diminishing the power of the circulation, should lead to a state of general cachexia, and how cachexia should lead to the deposition of tuberculous matter. But whether it be understood or not, it is a matter of fact that abdominal plethora is an almost constant concomitant of tuberculous cachexia. We are doubtless ignorant of many of the morbid conditions in the animal economy which combine to give a determinate effect to abdominal plethora; but the causes which are well known to give rise to the disordered state of health which precedes and leads to tuberculous cachexia, and the most successful means of correcting this, alike support our opinion of the presence of abdominal congestion, and afford a rational explanation of the phenomena of the disease.

Congestion of the venous system of the abdomen has long been regarded as a fruitful source of disease. It was familiar to the pathologists and physicians of the last century, and, although less attended to, has not been overlooked by the moderns. Such of my readers as are conversant with the writings of the German physicians of the middle of the last century, particularly Stahl,* Hoffmann,† and above all Kaempf and his disciples, will be aware of the extensive influence of this state of the abdominal circulation, and the importance attached to it at that time.‡ Referring to those works where the facts upon which the doctrine rests are fully exposed, I shall confine myself to a few remarks more particularly bearing upon my subject, and

---

* See his " Vena Portæ, Porta Malorum."

† Med. Rat. t. i. s. l. cap. viii.

‡ John Kaempf, the original improver, if not author, of this doctrine of *abdominal infarctus*, and of its peculiar treatment by clysters, did not himself publish any work on the subject. The doctrine was first made known in the inaugural dissertation of his eldest son, (also named John,) *De infarctu vasorum ventriculi*, published at Basil in 1751. It was afterwards more fully developed in the dissertation of Koch, *De infarctibus vasorum in infimo ventre*, Argent, 1752; of Schmid, *De concrementis uteri*, Basil, 1753; of Elvert, *De infarctibus venarum abdominalium*, Tubing. 1754; of Faber and Brotbeck, *Ulterior expositio novæ methodæ Kaempfianæ*, Tubing. 1755; of G. L. Kaempf, (the second son,) *De morbis ex atrophia*, Basil, 1756; and, finally, in the treatise published in his native language by John, the eldest son, entitled *Fur Aertze und Kranke bestimmte abhandlung, &c.* Dessau, 1784–8. The best of these dissertations, viz. those of J. Kaempf, Koch, Elvert, and Faber and Brotbeck, are reprinted in the third volume of *Baldinger's Syllogr*, Gott. 1778.

which it is but justice to myself to say were established in my mind, as the result, or supposed result,
of observation, before I became acquainted with
the German doctrines of abdominal infarctus.

Of the various phenomena presented by a person
strongly predisposed to or labouring under tuberculous disease, a congestive state of the abdominal
venous circulation will, I believe, be found, on close
investigation, to be one of the most constant. In
children, originally of a strumous habit, we observe
a constant disposition to this congestive state of the
abdominal circulation; and unless we succeed in
obviating it, they become tuberculous, and die
early in life. In youth we find the same state of
congestion as a precursor of tuberculous cachexia;
at this age it manifests itself often by epistaxis, by
hemoptysis, and even by hemorrhoids; but it is
during the middle period of life, from thirty-five
to fifty, that it is accompanied with more marked
symptoms, such as dyspepsia and its various con-
comitants, which exist often for a very considerable
time, and not unfrequently obscure the pulmonary
affection till tuberculous disease has made extensive progress.

Congestion and disordered function of the abdominal viscera have long been remarked as causes
of consumption : they were regarded by Kaempf
and his disciples as giving rise to most of the
chronic diseases of the chest. Portal and several

other foreign authors have also remarked the connexion of consumption with abdominal disease, but
in a manner so vague and undefined as to attract
little attention. In this country, likewise, several
authors have noticed the congestive state of the
abdominal circulation, more especially congestion
and deranged function of the liver, as a frequent
source of similar disease; among these authors
may be particularly mentioned Mr. Abernethy,*
Dr. Wilson Philip,† and Dr. Ayre;‡ and, more recently, Dr. Todd, in his comprehensive article on
" Indigestion," already referred to, has given in
his pathology of *strumous dyspepsia*, views corresponding exactly with those just stated. " The
phenomena of this disease," he observes, " its whole
complexion and character, sufficiently indicate a
congestive state of the hepatic system; and were
we to assume, as the proximate cause of the disease, a plethora of the vena portarum, both in its
roots and branches, we should be furnished with
the means of explaining all the symptoms of the
disease; for we should readily understand how, in
this state of the circulation of the abdomen, the
mucous surfaces of the intestines should be full of

* On the Constitutional Origin of Local Diseases.

† On " Indigestion" and on the " Influence of Minute Doses
of Mercury," &c.

‡ Practical Observations on the Nature and Treatment of Marasmus.

blood, consequently subject to inflammatory irrita-
tions and disordered functions, whilst the peculiar
office of the duodenum renders it specially liable
to be the seat of them : how the function of the
liver being deranged, all the other consequences
of this disease may follow : for though we may not
know precisely what share the functions of the
liver have in the process of sanguification, we
can easily understand how it may interrupt and
interfere with this process, leading to a cachectic
state of the fluids, from which result tubercles and
other semi-vital and semi-organic productions. Nor
does it seem an improbable supposition that a disposition to abdominal plethora, or an organization
which favours it, may be transmitted by parents to
their offspring, more especially in dyspeptic and
hypochondriacal persons, in whom the chylopoietic
viscera, under constant irritation, are necessarily
also in a state of congestion: we might thus explain
how the strumous cachexy is continued, and how it
is generated."*

The practice generally adopted in this country in
strumous diseases no doubt originated in the idea
that they were connected with hepatic congestion ;
but the harsh means employed to obviate it have
often proved more injurious than beneficial. This
has arisen chiefly from the nature of the affection

* Op. cit.

not being understood. With the hepatic and general abdominal congestion there is very generally combined irritation of the intestinal mucous surfaces, and the means often employed to relieve the one of these affections increase the other. The whole subject of abdominal plethora and gastrointestinal irritation has not yet been fully investigated, nor the influence of this pathological condition in the production of tuberculous disease well understood.

I do not, however, wish it to be inferred that I consider abdominal congestion as a pathological condition that must necessarily be followed by tuberculous disease. In strong and healthy constitutions nature has provided processes in the form of diseases for the relief of this morbid condition, of which gout, hemorrhoids, and cutaneous diseases offer the most ready examples. When nature or the constitution has not power to operate these corrective processes, that morbid condition is induced by abdominal plethora which leads to the formation of tubercles. The stronger children of gouty parents inherit the gout: the more weakly become tuberculous. In the history of the diseases of families, it is matter of common occurrence to observe the gouty constitution gradually degenerate into the tuberculous. On the other hand, neither do I mean to maintain that the morbid condition of body which precedes the formation of tubercles must necessarily be preceded by abdominal ple-thora. We can easily understand how that morbid condition may be brought about without the inter-vention of abdominal plethora. All I contend for is, that in the ordinary course of civilized life it is the most general mode by which tuberculous cachexia is induced, and on that account the most important to be known. Of the various other conditions of the system which may contribute to the production of tuberculous cachexia, little is known: I have already noticed as a very probable predisposing cause, a feeble heart,—a condition which a congestive state of the venous system tends strongly to augment.

CHAPTER XII.

UNDER the head of prevention, the first and most important inquiry which claims our attention involves the consideration of two distinct objects— the arresting the hereditary transmission of the disease, and the prevention of its developement in children born with the constitutional predisposition.

SECT. I.—PREVENTION AS REGARDS PARENTS.

When treating of the causes, I endeavoured to show that parents may transmit the tuberculous constitution to their children. Every member of the profession, by observing what is daily passing before him, may see numerous proofs of the truth of this statement: he will find many children presenting the tuberculous constitution, while no traces of this are to be observed in the parents. The children of those who have suffered long from dyspeptic complaints, gout, cutaneous affections, or any other form of chronic disease originating in derangement of the digestive function, which has produced an influence on the constitution, are very frequently the subjects of scrofula, or of disorders which dispose to and ultimately induce tuberculous cachexia.

In order, therefore, effectually to prevent the extension of tuberculous disease, we must in the first place direct our attention to the state of the parents. Were parents in general convinced that the health of their children depended chiefly upon the integrity of their own health, a beneficial effect might be produced upon society at large, and especially on the members of strumous families. If a more healthy and natural mode of living were adopted by persons in that rank of life which gives them the power of choice, and if more consideration were bestowed on matrimonial alliances, the disease which is so often entailed on their offspring might not only be prevented, but even the predisposition to it extinguished in their families, in the course of a few generations. In the present state of society, it is needless to observe that the reverse of this very commonly happens ; and from the total disregard of the circumstances alluded to, the race often terminates in the third generation. The children of dyspeptic persons generally become the subjects of dyspepsia in a greater degree and at an earlier age than their parents ; and if they marry into families of a strumous constitution, their offspring are frequently found to be scrofulous and to die of consumption, or some other tuberculous diseases, in early youth, and even in infancy. I could adduce many melancholy examples of the truth of this observation ; but it is at least consolatory to know that the evil may be obviated ; and it is a duty which parents owe to their offspring to endeavour to correct it.

Members of families already predisposed to tuberculous disease should at least endeavour to avoid matrimonial alliances with others in the same condition ; but above all they should avoid the too common practice of intermarrying among their own immediate relatives,—a practice at once a fertile source of scrofula, a sure mode of deteriorating the intellectual and physical powers, and eventually the means of extinguishing a degenerated race. "There can be no question," says Dr. Mason Good, " that inter-marriages, among the collateral branches of the same family, tend more than any thing else to fix and multiply, and aggravate hereditary predisposition. And hence, nothing can be wiser, on physical as well as on moral grounds, than the restraints which divine and human laws have concurred in laying on marriages between relations."*

* Study of Medicine, vol. v. p. 35.

It would also be well if persons contemplating mar-
riage were aware of the necessity of attending to
their health, previously to, and after the adoption
of this change of life. The dyspeptic should have
recourse to such means as would restore the functions of his digestive organs, and should adopt and
adhere to a regimen calculated to prevent the recurrence of his complaint; the gouty subject
should renounce the well-known causes of his disorder; but those who are afflicted with organic
disease, more especially with consumption, should
pause before they enter in a contract which can
only entail disease or unhappiness on all concerned.

The full extent of misery arising from injudicious
marriages of this description is comprehended by
the medical practitioner only; he will, therefore,
appreciate the justness of these remarks, although he
will acknowledge the difficulty of enforcing the necessary restrictions on the practical consideration of
the public. I am well aware that mankind in
general are far too reckless to attend to any precautionary measures on this subject, even although
perfectly satisfied of their expediency; still there
is a small proportion, in that rank of life to which
the above remarks apply with the greatest force,
on whom these cautions may not be wholly thrown
away.

PREGNANCY. — Too little regard is paid by
females to their health during pregnancy, and they
are in general little aware of the influence which
their mode of living during this most important
period has upon their offspring. There are certain
rules of management and conduct which it is necessary for every mother to adopt at this time, and it
should be impressed upon the mind of the young
mother more especially, that, as her infant's health
mainly depends upon her attention to her own from
the commencement of this state, a great degree of
responsibility attaches to her. She should not for
a moment forget during her pregnancy that she is
a mother, and that whatever mode of living is most
conducive to her own health is the best guarantee
for that of her infant: if she is a member of a
delicate family, she should regard her health with
more than common solicitude.

It is a common opinion that during pregnancy
females require a fuller and more stimulating diet
than that to which they have been accustomed.
As a general rule this is a great error: the system
of a pregnant female acquires increased activity,
which, far from demanding increase of diet, renders
it often necessary to adopt a less exciting regimen,
especially in the advanced months, when stimulants
of all kinds are generally injurious. The more
plain and simple the diet, and the more sparingly

stimulants of all kinds are used, so much the better for both mother and child.

Daily exercise in the open air, suited to the strength of the individual, will be of the utmost advantage; and when circumstances permit, I would strongly recommend that the period of pregnancy should be passed in the country. Crowded assemblies of all kinds, public spectacles and theatrical exhibitions,—every thing, in short, calculated to excite strong feelings, to depress the mind, or rouse the passions, ought to be sedulously avoided.

There are numerous other circumstances regarding the conduct of females during pregnancy, which, as it more immediately devolves upon the medical attendant to point them out and to direct their application to individual cases, it would be superfluous to detail.

SECT. II.—PREVENTION AS REGARDS CHILDREN.

Although we are not acquainted with any direct means of correcting the constitutional predisposition to tuberculous disease, there can be no doubt that in many instances we have the power of effecting it indirectly.

By placing the predisposed child in the most favourable circumstances as regards those agents which exert a constant influence on the health, such as food, air, exercise, &c.,—by removing functional derangements as they occur, and especially by maintaining the digestive organs in a state of integrity, we may improve the constitution so as to enable it to overcome the hereditary predisposition. By the judicious adaptation of these means, I am persuaded that the lives of a large proportion of children, born with the predisposition, might be saved; and it is perhaps not beyond the truth to say that under the present system of management five-sixths perish.

In proceeding to develope more fully the measures which are deemed essential to the accomplishment of this object, I am well aware that many of my recommendations will unfortunately be found beyond the attainment of the public at large; but nevertheless I feel called upon to state them, in order that they may be adopted when circumstances admit of their application.

With the view of rendering my observations more practical, even at the risk of some repetition, I shall apply them to the different periods of life,—*infancy*, *childhood*, and *youth*; an arrangement of the subject highly important in treating of a disease the causes and remedies of which vary at different ages.

PREVENTION OF THE DISEASE IN INFANCY.

The rules for promoting the health of strumous infants are nearly the same as for others, but they require to be more rigidly enforced and more strictly adhered to. Unless the children of unhealthy parents be reared with the greatest attention to every circumstance which can contribute to health, they have little chance of reaching maturity without becoming the subjects of tuberculous disease.

Food, clothing, dress, bathing, air, and residence of infants.

Suckling.—If the infant derives the strumous constitution from both parents, or from the mother only, it should be suckled by a young healthy nurse; but should the disposition to disease be derived entirely from the father, and the mother's health be unexceptionable, she should suckle her own child. It is always satisfactory when this can be accomplished, as it is, with few exceptions, the plan most agreeable to the mother as well as most beneficial to her own health; and, if her mode of living be consistent with her duties as a nurse, it will be far better for the infant; but all these contingencies require consideration before we decide on the plan which it is most desirable to adopt when we are consulted in any particular case. I do not enter upon the moral consideration of this question,—I speak of it merely in a medical point of view; and I am satisfied that when the mother's health renders her unfit to nurse her child, or her

habits or mode of living are such as to prevent her
from adhering to those regulations by which every
nurse, whether mother or not, should abide, it is much
better for the health of the infant that it should derive
its first nourishment from the breast of a stranger.

The arguments advanced in favour of the opinion
that every mother should suckle her own infant,
appear plausible, and would be perfectly just if
every mother enjoyed that state of health which
renders her fit for such a duty. In the present
state of society, however, this is far from being
the case, and I therefore consider it better for the
delicate mother herself, and infinitely so for her
child, that she should at once renounce a task for
which her constitution renders her unfit, than
struggle on for a few months in an attempt which
may injure her own health and destroy her infant.
Half measures, so often recommended in such cases,
are always unwise; they generally end in the child
being fed by hand in place of being suckled,—a
plan which never fails, I believe, to injure the health
of the infant. I would therefore lay it down as a
rule, which should not be deviated from, when
circumstances admit of an adherence to it, that the
child of a consumptive mother, or of one in whom
the strumous constitution is strongly marked, should
be suckled by another woman, and that the period
of nursing should generally extend from twelve to
eighteen months, or even longer. I recommend

the suckling to be continued for this length of time, with a view to enable the infant to pass over the period of teething with greater safety : indeed the strumous infant should not be weaned till the first set of teeth have appeared ; it should have no food in general but the nurse's milk till six months old, and for some time after the food should be of the lightest quality, and constitute only a small proportion of the nutriment. I am aware that a difference of opinion may exist among medical men on the propriety of continuing to nourish the infant so long on the milk of the nurse alone, and that the good effects which have been obtained from feeding infants on animal broths may be cited against it; but it should be recollected that the experiments in support of this practice were made on children in foundling hospitals and other charitable institutions, where the suckling was very deficient. The milk of a healthy nurse constitutes, I believe, the most nutritious food for the infant during the first six months of its existence,—is the best adapted to the digestive organs, and supplies the elements of nutrition in the form and proportion most suitable to the organization of the infant.

It is almost unnecessary to add to these remarks that the selection of a nurse for an infant of strumous or delicate parents, deserves especial attention. She should be young, healthy, and free from all appearance of struma, and her own child should not be older than that which she is to suckle. She should take daily exercise in the open air; her regimen should not differ much from that to which she has been accustomed, or, if any change is made in it, it should be gradual and moderate. It is erroneous to suppose that women when nursing ought to be much more highly fed than at other times : a good nurse does not require such artificial aid, and a bad one will not be improved by it. The quantity and variety of food and liquids of an exciting quality, which many nurses consume, and the indolent life they too often lead, have invariably the effect of deranging the digestive organs, and induce a state of febrile excitement, or a premature return of the catamenia; circumstances which rarely fail to produce an injurious effect upon the health of the child.

Clothing.—The dress from birth should be loose, so as to admit of the free exercise of the limbs, and in point of warmth it should be carefully suited to the season. The whole surface, particularly the extremities, ought to be well protected during cold weather : the opinion that infants may be hardened by exposing them to the cold air in a half-covered state is erroneous in all cases, and in children of a delicate constitution leads to the most pernicious consequences.

Bathing.—The object of bathing children is two-fold ; the first and most important is cleanliness, which is peculiarly necessary in children of a strumous constitution, as in them the cutaneous secretions are rarely in a healthy proportion. At first the infant should be washed with warm water; and for this purpose a bath in which it may be immersed every night, with the view of thoroughly cleaning the whole surface, will be beneficial; by degrees the water with which it is sponged in the morning may be made tepid, but the night bath should be continued of a temperature grateful to the feelings. The second object in bathing being to brace and strengthen, the child may, as it increases in age, be sponged with cold water, or even plunged into it with advantage every morning during the summer. Much has been said and written in favour of cold bathing; and the authors who have laid down rules on this subject have been fond of adducing in support of the practice the customs of savage nations, altogether overlooking the difference in the condition of infants in civilised life. Unquestionably the judicious adoption of cold sponging and bathing, with subsequent friction of the body with flannel, is one of the most effectual means of strengthening children; but its effects must be carefully watched, as all will not be equally benefited, and the health of some may even be injured by it.

Air.—As the respiration of an impure atmosphere is one of the most powerful causes of tuberculous cachexia, so is the respiration of pure air an indispensable requisite for strumous children; indeed, without this all our efforts to improve their health will fail. Too much attention, therefore, cannot be paid to the construction and ventilation of the child's apartments : the room in which he sleeps should be large, the air should be frequently renewed, and his bed should not have more curtains than are necessary to protect him from currents of air. The custom which prevails in this country of surrounding beds with thick curtains is most injurious to health ; and it is to this habit, and to the heated atmosphere of their bed-rooms, that the languor and bloated appearance of many young persons, on first awaking in the morning, are in a great measure to be attributed. Bed-rooms ought to be large in all their dimensions, they should be in an elevated part of the house, and so situated as to admit a free supply both of air and light : those apartments to which the sun's rays and the refreshing breeze have free access, are always.the most healthy and desirable. These remarks are applicable to all apartments, but they deserve especial attention in those of infants, and young children, on account of their being necessarily so much confined to them.

The proper time for carrying an infant into the open air must be determined by the season of the year and the state of the weather. A delicate in-

fant born late in the autumn will not generally
derive advantage from being carried into the open
air, in this climate, till the succeeding spring; and
if the rooms in which he is kept are large and well
ventilated, he will not suffer from the confinement,
while he will most probably escape catarrhal affections, which so often result from the injudicious
exposure of infants to a cold or humid atmosphere.

Residence.—It is almost unnecessary to say, that
when an infant can be suckled in a healthy situation
in the country, it is, *cæteris paribus*, far preferable
to the town ; but the choice of situation is generally
so little regarded, and yet requires so much judgment,
that I may be excused for offering a few remarks on
the rules by which it should be regulated.

There is no circumstance connected with health,
concerning which the public are, in my opinion, so
ill informed, as the requisites of a healthy residence, both as regards local position and internal
construction. In this island we have chiefly to
guard against humidity, on which account our
houses should not be built in low, confined situations, nor too near water, especially when stagnant,
and, still less, near marshes. Neither should a
house be too closely surrounded by trees or shrubs.
Trees at some distance from a house are both an
ornament and an advantage, but become injurious
when so near as to overshadow it, or prevent the

air from circulating freely around it and through its various apartments. The atmosphere of a building overhung by trees, or surrounded by a thick shrubbery, is kept in a state of constant humidity, except in the driest weather; and the health of the inmates rarely fails to suffer in consequence. The natural moisture of the country arising from the humid state of the soil and luxuriant vegetation, is greatly increased by such an injudicious mode of planting; an artificial atmosphere being created, which renders a situation of this kind less healthy than the more open parts of large towns. It is not generally known how limited may be the range of a damp unhealthy atmosphere; a low shaded situation may be capable of inducing tuberculous disease in an infant, while a rising ground a few hundred yards distant may afford a healthy site for his residence. The dryness of the air in towns, which is the consequence of good drainage and an artificial soil, is at once the safeguard of the inhabitants, and a compensation, in some measure, for the want of that unimpeded circulation and renewal of pure air which the country alone affords.

I have been led to make these remarks while treating of infants, because, from being necessarily much confined to the house, they suffer more from the causes which have been noticed. The health of females, also, and for the same reason, is more injured than that of the male inhabitants, who pass much of their time in the open air.*

PREVENTION OF THE DISEASE IN CHILDHOOD.

During the period of childhood the same unremitting attention to the principal circumstances mentioned under the head of infancy is necessary. The important process of teething being accomplished, and the child having acquired the means of masticating, the food may be of a more substantial kind, but it must be carefully regulated by the powers of the digestive organs and by the constitution. In proportion to the delicacy of the child, the diet will in general require to be mild;

---

* It would be well if architects were to make themselves acquainted with the circumstances which contribute most essentially to the salubrity of habitations, as regards the site, the exposure, the drainage, and the size and disposition of the rooms. In many houses, in other respects well proportioned and arranged, the want of height in the bed-rooms is, I am persuaded, the cause of much ill-health. In our small country-houses this fault is very conspicuous; and the country-houses of our gentry are in many instances rendered unhealthy for one half of the year by the nature of the situation in which they are built, and this is frequently the case, too, when unexceptionable sites are to be found in the immediate vicinity. Numerous elegant buildings around this metropolis are more unhealthy than the central parts of the city, from the same causes. The evil consequences of inattention to these circumstances are experienced in all classes of habitations from the palace to the cottage.

while he thrives upon farinaceous food, milk and light broths, no stronger or more substantial diet need be used during the first two years : when he looks healthy, and grows, and his bowels are regular, (for this is one of the surest indications that the food is suited to the digestive organs,) we have the best proofs that the diet agrees with him.* When, on the other hand, the child appears heated or flushed towards evening, drinks greedily, and more than is usual in children of the same age, and when the bowels do not act regularly, we may be assured that there is something wrong in the regimen, or some derangement in the functions of the digestive organs, which requires immediate attention. There is no greater error in the management of children than that of giving them animal diet very early. To feed an infant with solid animal food before it has teeth proper for masticating, shows a total disregard to the plain

---

* I am glad to be able to cite the late Dr. Pemberton in support of the advantages of long suckling and a mild diet : " If a child is born of scrofulous parents, I would strongly recommend that it be entirely nourished from the breast of a healthy nurse for at least a year ; after this the food should consist of milk and farinaceous vegetables. By a perseverance in this diet for three years, I have imagined that the threatened scrofulous appearances have certainly been postponed, if not altogether prevented." *A Practical Treatise on various Diseases of the Abdominal Viscera*, by C. R. Pemberton, M.D., F.R.S., &c. p. 201, second edition.

indications of nature in withholding teeth suited to this purpose, until the age at which the system requires solid food. Before that time, milk, farinaceous food, and animal broths afford that kind of sustenance which is at once best suited to the digestive organs and to the nutrition of the system. The method of mincing and pounding meat as a substitute for mastication, may do very well for the toothless octogenarian, whose stomach has been habituated to concentrated nutriment; but the digestive organs of a child are not adapted to the due preparation of such food, and will be disordered by it. When the child has the means of masticating, a little animal food may be allowed; but at first this should be of the lightest quality, and allowed on alternate days only, and even then its effects should be watched; for all changes in the regimen of children should be gradual.

The observation of the frequent origin of scrofulous disease in defective nourishment, has led to the opposite extreme of overfeeding; and children who are disposed to tuberculous disease are too often put upon a regimen which favours the development of the disease which it is intended to prevent. By persevering in the use of an overstimulating diet the digestive organs become irritated, and the various secretions immediately connected with and necessary to digestion are diminished, especially the biliary secretion; at least the sensible qualities of the bile enable us better to observe its changes. Constipation of the bowels and congestion of the abdominal circulation succeed, followed by the train of consequences which have already been detailed. Children so fed become, moreover, very liable to attacks of fever, and of inflammation, affecting particularly the mucous membranes; and measles and the other diseases incident to childhood are generally severe in their attack.

Exercise.—When the child has acquired sufficient strength to take active exercise, he can scarcely be too much in the open air; the more he is accustomed to it, the more capable will he be of bearing the vicissitudes of the climate. If children are allowed to amuse themselves at pleasure, they will generally take that kind and degree of exercise which is best calculated to promote the growth and development of the body. When they are too feeble to take sufficient exercise on foot, riding on a donkey or pony forms the best substitute: this kind of exercise is at all times of infinite service to delicate children; it amuses the mind and exercises the muscles of the whole body, and in so gentle a manner as to induce little fatigue. Young girls should be allowed and even encouraged to take the same kinds of exercise as boys: it is chiefly the unrestrained freedom of active play that renders them so much less subject to curvatures of the spine and other deformities than girls,—a large proportion of whom are more or less mishapen, in consequence of the unnatural restraint which is imposed upon them by their dress and imperfect exercise.

The clothing of young persons requires particular attention, and must of course be regulated according to the season. The winter dress should be resumed early and laid aside late in the spring. In spring and autumn the vicissitudes of our climate are greatest, and congestive and inflammatory affections most common: this is peculiarly the case in the spring, which is also the season when local strumous affections are most liable to occur in constitutions disposed to them. Flannel next the skin is not only proper but generally necessary; cotton may be substituted during the summer, the flannel being resumed early in the autumn: it may be put off with advantage during the night.

Education.—The education of strumous children requires much judgment and consideration; no child should be condemned to pass the greater part of the day in the close apartments of a crowded school until he has attained his ninth year at least.

The period of confinement in schools is much too long for the health of all children, and might be abridged not only without detriment but with advantage to their instruction: the young mind is

easily wearied, and it is not sufficiently considered
that the development of the intellectual powers
ought for a time to give way, in delicate children,
to the physical improvement of the general system.

The situation and construction of the school
should be free from all the objections which I
have already pointed out, when noticing the causes
of unhealthiness in country residences. School-
rooms ought to be large and lofty, so as to admit
of free ventilation without the risk of exposure to
currents of cold air. The impure atmosphere which
too commonly prevails in schools is an unfailing
source of injury to health. During the first years
of education, children should be allowed a little
relaxation and play in the open air when the weather permits, at intervals during the school hours.
At no period of youth should education be pushed
beyond its proper limits, or the mind be worked
above its powers; the welfare of the pupil demands
the observance of this rule on the part of the
master as well as the parents, more especially when
the child belongs to that class of strumous children
whose intellects are preternaturally acute. Unfortunately, however, these are generally the pupils
selected by the master to do credit to his establishment; every means are taken to encourage this
premature manifestation of mind, and to stimulate
the child to renewed exertions; and thus the health
is enfeebled, and even life is often sacrificed at a

period of brilliant promise, when the hopes of friends are buoyed up by fallacious expectations, which a more rational system of education might have realized.

In some cases, the mischief resulting from this cause makes its appearance at an early age; in other instances, not till towards the period of puberty. I have met with many distressing examples of young men, who, after years of close application at school, had entered upon their studies at the university with the same unabated zeal, but who were soon compelled, by the sudden failure of their health, to abandon their literary pursuits and the prospects which they had in view, with their constitutions permanently injured. No subject, I am persuaded, calls more urgently for the attention of parents than the education of their children, both intellectual and physical. However laudable may be their desire to see the minds of their offspring early and highly cultivated, it should be checked by the knowledge that this object can in many cases be attained only by the sacrifice of health, and too often not without the loss of life. " The time," says Dr. Beddoes, " is not perhaps far distant when parents shall discover that the best method of cultivating the understanding, provides at the same time most effectually for robustness of constitution; and that the means of securing both parts of the comprehensive prayer of the

U

satirist,—*ut sit mens sana in corpore sano*—are identical."

The consequences just noticed as arising from the erroneous system of education in the schools for boys, prevail in a greater degree, and are productive of more injury, in female boarding-schools. If the plans pursued at many of these establishments were intended to injure the health of the pupils, they could scarcely be better contrived to effect that purpose. The prevailing system of female education is, indeed, fraught with the most pernicious consequences. At a period of life when the development of the system demands the most judicious management, young girls are sent to schools where almost the only object which appears to claim consideration, is the amount of mental improvement, or rather the variety of accomplishments with which they can be stored. At an early hour in the morning the pupil is set down to music or the drawing-table, where she remains, often in a constrained position, in a cold room, till the whole frame, and more especially the lower extremities, become chilled :—the brief relaxation during the short space allowed for meals and the formal walk, is insufficient to restore the natural warmth of the extremities ; and it often happens that girls are allowed to retire to bed with their feet so cold as frequently to prevent sleep for hours. Those who are acquainted with the general system of the boarding-schools of this country will allow that this is no exaggerated picture.* A delicate girl submitted to such a discipline cannot escape disease. While school-boys have the advantage of a play-ground, or enjoy their recreation at pleasure in the open fields, the unfortunate inmates of a female boarding-school are only permitted to walk along the foot-paths in pairs, in stiff and monotonous formality, resembling, as Beddoes justly remarks, a funeral procession. The consequence is, that the muscles of the upper extremities and those which are chiefly concerned in the support of the trunk are rarely called into active play; they do not acquire strength as the body increases in stature,--they remain weak and unequal to the task of supporting the trunk in the erect posture. A curved state of the spine is generally the consequence; and this, by altering the natural position and form of the trunk, renders the respiratory movements imperfect; the capacity of the chest is diminished, and the lungs are consequently more liable to congestion, and the diseases which are its consequences.

While the natural form and proportions of the body are thus destroyed, the health generally suffers in a remarkable manner. This is generally manifested

* See the excellent article on PHYSICAL EDUCATION, by Dr. Barlow of Bath, in the *Cyclopædia of Practical Medicine*.

by the paleness of the countenance, by a deranged state of the digestive organs, by a dry coarse skin, cutaneous eruptions, and other indications of dete- riorated health. In short, almost all the requisites for the production of scrofula may be found in female boarding-schools, where the system I have described is pursued.

There are many exceptions to this system of boarding-school discipline, and the number would no doubt be greatly increased if the conductors were aware of one-half of the extent of the inju- rious effects it produces. In the establishments to which I allude, as being conducted on more rational principles, the cultivation of the mind and the ac- quirement of the various female accomplishments are not the only objects aimed at; the health of the girls forms, as it ought, the first and paramount consideration. The time devoted to daily study by the present system should be greatly abridged, and that allowed for exercise augmented in proportion ; the exercise should also be such as to call into action every muscle of the body.

The clothing during the winter ought to be warm, and every means should be adopted to guard against coldness of the extremities. The pupils should not be allowed to sit so long at one time as to induce this state, nor to go to bed with chilled feet. Were I to select any one circumstance more injurious than another to the health of young girls, it would be cold extremities, the consequence of want of active exercise, and the prevailing and most pernicious habit of wearing thin shoes while in the house.

A warm bath ought to form an appendage to every boarding-school, and every girl should occasionally enjoy the benefit of it. A large, lofty, and well-ventilated room should be set apart for the express purpose of exercise, when the weather is such as to prevent it in the open air. A system of gymnastics is quite as necessary for girls as for boys. They should be sufficiently varied to give free play to all the muscles, and more especially to those of the trunk and upper extremities. If the girl has any tendency to curvature of the spine, those exercises which are most effectual in correcting this deformity should constitute a part of the daily exercise. To the room devoted to these exercises, the younger girls should be allowed to retire for a short time, during the usual hours of school, to amuse themselves at pleasure. This recreation I consider of the utmost importance: it must, nevertheless, be understood that no exercise is to be considered a substitute for that in the open air; and for this reason every female boarding-school ought to have a play-ground, where the pupils may choose their own amusements and play without restraint.

Were a judicious system of management pur-

sued in boarding-schools, the opprobrium which
has so long attached to them, would not only be
removed, but they might be made the means of
improving the general health of the pupils, and of
correcting even the scrofulous constitution; they
would thus become the source of much future
benefit to the children and of happiness to their
parents.

It is almost unnecessary to observe that all tight
dressing is utterly incompatible with the extent and
variety of exercise which has been recommended,
and ought, therefore, to be discarded. The idea
that young females require *stays* as a means of
support is admitted by all medical men to be most
erroneous; such mechanical restraint to the free
motions of the trunk of the growing female is productive of much evil and frequent deformity. If
girls were strengthened by the various means which
are within the reach of all, and which nature points
out to us as best, such artificial support would not
be necessary before maturity, and even then would
be scarcely wanted.

When we take a comprehensive view of the
nature and causes of tuberculous diseases generally,
the claim which the present subject has upon our
best attention must be apparent; and in urging it
on the consideration of the profession, I would beg
to remind them that it is chiefly through their exer-

tions that the desired improvements can be effected. It is during the period of youth only, that the constitutional tendency to these destructive diseases can be corrected, and to effect this, as Beddoes justly remarks, is unquestionably the most important object of physical education.

PREVENTION OF THE DISEASE IN YOUTH.

The period of life which extends from youth to adult age, from about the eighteenth to the twenty-fifth year in males, and the sixteenth to the twenty-second in females, is one of great importance as regards persons predisposed to consumption. If the health has suffered by mismanagement in education, or from other causes, during early youth, the system very often shows it in a remarkable manner about the period of puberty. The development of the body which should naturally take place at this age, and which in healthy persons is accompanied with an increase of strength and vigour in the system, is often delayed beyond the usual period, or imperfectly accomplished. If, therefore, young persons remain weak and thin, or look unhealthy after the usual period of puberty, they may be considered in great danger of falling into tuberculous cachexia. Those who have been over-worked at school, or kept much at sedentary occupations, frequently present this state of deteriorated health.

Under such circumstances, the utmost care will be necessary to prevent tuberculous disease. A strict examination and inquiry should be made into the state of every function, and more especially of those connected with nutrition. The condition of the digestive organs and skin requires particular attention, because they are most commonly deranged : the tongue will very often be found furred ; the alvine evacuations irregular ; and the skin dry, harsh, and affected with eruptions, particularly with *acne* in its various forms : in young females the catamenia are retarded, or imperfectly established. Such are the common symptoms presented to us in these cases, but they admit of considerable variety in different constitutions and temperaments.

The absolute necessity of early attention to these indications of tuberculous cachexia cannot be too strongly impressed by medical men upon the minds of parents. There can be no doubt that a very large proportion of our youth who fall victims to consumption from twenty to thirty years of age, might be saved by a timely adoption of the simple measures detailed in this chapter, and which are, in some degree, within the power and reach of all.

In the deranged condition of health to which I refer, the pulse is generally feeble ; the venous system is overcharged ; and the change in the balance between the arterial and venous circulation, which usually occurs only after the middle period of life, takes place in such persons before they have reached maturity, and hence we find an explanation of some of their diseases. The chief object in our preventive treatment ought to be the maintenance of a healthy condition of the chylopoietic system, and an active state of the pulmonary and cutaneous functions; for which purpose very simple and available remedies are generally found sufficient:— exercise in the open air, and above all on horseback, warm bathing, friction of the surface, and proper clothing, along with a residence in a healthy part of the country, will often, in a few months, produce the most beneficial change on such constitutions.

There is one kind of exercise which has not been sufficiently attended to in the prevention of pulmonary disease, but which deserves particular notice in this place; I allude to the exercise of the respiratory organs, and of all the muscles employed in the process of respiration. The great object of such exercise is to ensure the due proportions of the chest and the free and full action of the lungs.

Dr. Autenrieth, of Tubingen, according to Sir Alexander Crichton, first recommended the practice of improving the narrow and contracted chest by deep and frequent inspirations. He advised his patients to place their hands upon some solid support, and to exercise themselves by taking repeated deep inspirations; but cautioned them against carrying this so far as to produce pain.* I have been in the habit of recommending the full expansion of the chest, desiring young persons, while standing, to throw the arms and shoulders back, and while in this position, to inhale slowly as much air as they can, and repeat this exercise at short intervals several times in succession: when this can be done in the open air, it is most desirable, a double advantage being obtained from the practice. Some exercise of this kind should be adopted daily by all young persons, more especially by those whose chests are narrow or deformed. Fencing, the use of dumb bells, and similar modes of exercising the arms, are also eminently useful in attaining the important end we have in view,—the full development of the chest and upper extremities; but they should never be carried so far as to induce fatigue or uneasiness.

Of the various modes of exercising the muscles of the trunk and upper extremities, the method which is employed in the army, as a preparation for the sword exercise, appears to me the best, and most generally applicable. It is called the club exercise, from the circumstance of two long pieces of wood, or clubs, being the weights employed. The clubs vary in weight according to the strength of the individual who is to use them. The person

* Crichton, op. cit. p. 137.

standing upright with a club in each hand, passes
them alternately over the head and round the shoulders in various ways so as to call into successive or
combined action the whole muscles of the arms and
trunk. The action is not violent, but rather gentle
and steady, and in this respect the clubs are superior to dumb bells. The practice is borrowed
from the Persians and Hindoos, who carry it to a
much greater extent than has been attempted in
this country, and with the effect of producing a remarkable development of the muscles of the trunk
and arms, with a corresponding increase of strength.
This mode of exercise is admirably suited for an in-
door exercise to young persons of both sexes. It is
especially useful to girls, who, without some artificial exercise of this kind, rarely have the muscles
of the chest and back sufficiently called into action.
The daily use of the clubs would contribute more
to the proper development of the chest, and to give
a straight back and a good figure, than all the lessons of the dancing-master. All persons engaged
in the education or direction of youth, should make
themselves acquainted with this mode of exercise ;
every school and family should be provided with
sets of clubs suited to the age and strength of the
children : a few lessons would be sufficient to in-
struct any person in this admirable exercise. If
such exercises as have been noticed were regularly
employed under proper restrictions, they would not

merely favour the full proportions of the chest, but
would tend also to obviate the disproportion between the upper and lower extremities which we so
frequently observe in youth, and which is evidently
the consequence of defective exercise of the former.
I also consider exercises of this description very
useful to persons confined to the desk, or engaged in
occupations which require a bent or stooping posture, by which the free expansion of the chest is impeded; and especially to those mechanics, whose
constrained position seldom allows the upper parts
of the chest to be fully expanded. The comparative
immobility of the upper parts of the lung is probably
a chief cause of their being much more frequently
the seat of tuberculous disease, than the lower and
more moveable portions. " If we compare," observes
Dr. Carswell, " the functional activity, or, rather,
the extent of mobility possessed by the inferior and
superior lobes of the lungs, we at once perceive a
most remarkable difference in favour of the former.
The inferior lobe ascends and descends throughout
a space equal to that to which the diaphragm is capable of contracting, and expands in all directions
to the fullest extent of the dilated inferior walls of
the thorax. The upper lobe, on the contrary, has
hardly any motion of ascent and descent, and a very
limited lateral expansion. Under these circumstances, what should be the effect produced on a
substance such as tuberculous matter effused into

the vesicular structure of these two lobes? In the former we should naturally expect that there would be a continual tendency towards the expulsion of this matter, whilst in the latter there would be the same tendency to its accumulation. May it not be owing to the facility with which the tuberculous matter escapes, that we do not find it accumulated on the mucous surface of the larger bronchi, or of the trachea, or on that of the intestines?"

Reading aloud and public recitation will, also, when prudently employed, be useful in strengthening both the pulmonary and digestive organs, and in giving tone and power to the voice. The clear and distinct enunciation which is acquired by long practice only, is seldom found associated with pulmonary disease, and I therefore commend the practice of recitation and elocution at schools.

The modes of exercising the pulmonary organs which I have just described are equally useful and more necessary to young females. The club exercise is particularly suited to them; and the ancient and well-known game of battle-dore and shuttlecock is one of the very best exercises for girls within doors.

I would not have it implied by these observations on the utility of exercising the respiratory muscles, that I consider a narrow chest the cause of consumption; but I do consider it important that the capacity of the chest should bear its full proportion to the other organs, and to the general development of the body; whenever this is not the case, the respiratory functions are less perfectly performed, and sanguification is impeded, while the lungs are more liable to congestion, a condition favourable to tuberculous and other diseases. In this way a diminutive capacity of the chest predisposes to tuberculous disease of the lungs; while a large and well-formed chest is unfavourable to them. Dr. Carswell justly remarks, " Whatever kind of employment or mode of life necessitates or facilitates an ample display and active state of the respiratory organs, is generally admitted as a powerful means of preventing the occurrence of tubercular phthisis. We are far from believing that such prophylactic means operate merely on the mechanical principle of the localization of the tuberculous deposition in the lungs, inasmuch as when these organs are placed under the favourable conditions just mentioned, the circulation, nutrition, secretion, and innervation of the same organs must acquire a vigour and harmony of action which will render them the least apt to receive or retain any morbid impression or change whatever."

But while I so highly approve of these exercises, I would strongly condemn those which require excessive bodily exertion, such as climbing precipices, &c., and which have been sometimes recommended for the prevention of consumption. Such violent efforts undoubtedly exercise the lungs, but they at the same time excite an inordinate action of the heart, and render it liable to be oppressed by the blood being suddenly forced upon it by the excessive muscular contractions. I consider all such violent exertion fraught with danger: indeed I have met with several cases of dilated heart in young persons, apparently originating in forcible and long-continued exertion, as in boat-rowing, &c.

But of all kinds of exercise, that which I consider the most advantageous to young persons of both sexes, and more especially to boys, is riding on horseback. No other exercise calls the whole muscles into such general action without fatigue; it promotes a free circulation in the surface and extremities, and the full play of the respiratory organs. The free exposure also to the pure air, which such exercise necessarily implies, contributes greatly to the advantage derived from it. Delicate children, or those hereditarily predisposed to consumptive disease, should, when it can be done, be taught to ride early. This ought to form part of the daily exercise, when the state of the weather does not forbid, and should be carried to a greater extent than it usually is, when adopted with the view of strengthening delicate children and young persons.

There are also other rules relating to this important period of life which the medical attendant will not fail to keep in mind in laying down direc-

tions for his youthful patient; but these are so
obvious that it is unnecessary to enter on them.*

* I have great pleasure and satisfaction in referring the general
as well as medical reader to the excellent work of Dr. Coombe,
for much valuable information on the subject of this chapter, as
well as on other points regarding the means of preserving and
improving the health.(1)   The circumstance of this valuable work
having reached a third edition in less than one year, is at once a
proof of its excellence and of the increasing desire for useful
knowledge in the public.

Since the publication of Dr. Coombe's work, several others
have appeared on the same subject, though differing somewhat in
plan.   Among these deserve to be particularly mentioned the
popular and very useful work of Dr. Hodgkin,(2) and that of
Dr. Southwood Smith.(3)

There is no subject more deserving of general study, and none
with which the public is less acquainted, than the means of preserving and improving the health.   The works to which I have
referred will be productive of much benefit to the rising generation, and deserve to be generally known and read.   They should
be in the hands of every person engaged in the education or
direction of youth.

In America the subject is also attracting attention.   Dr. Coombe's
work has been stereotyped there, and I have just received a comprehensive work on Hygiene by Dr. Dunglisson, Professor of
Hygiene, &c., in the University of Baltimore.

(1) *The Principles of Physiology applied to the Preservation of Health,
and to the Improvement of Physical and Mental Education.*   Third edition,
1835.

(2) *Lectures on the Means of Promoting and Preserving Health.* 1835.

(3) *The Philosophy of Health.* 1835.

(4) *Elements of Hygiene.* 1835.

In concluding these remarks on the means of preserving health and preventing tuberculous diseases, I would advert to a circumstance of great importance,—the choice of a profession. This is a subject which is much neglected, and hence the unhappy results which so frequently ensue from the ill-judged selection of professions without any regard to health. It is most essential that the parent, in selecting a profession for his son, should consider well whether his physical powers are sufficient to sustain the duties inseparable from it. In all ranks of life much might be done to preserve the health by choosing occupations suited to individual constitutions.

CHAPTER XIII.

TREATMENT OF TUBERCULOUS CACHEXIA.

HAVING, in an early part of this work (Chapter II.), endeavoured to describe the characteristic features of the tuberculous constitution and tuberculous cachexia, I would simply observe, in entering upon the subject of Treatment, that a familiar acquaintance with these characters is most essential to the practitioner, inasmuch as it will assist him greatly in forming a correct judgment of the case, more especially when the signs of local disease are equivocal or obscure.

The correction of the constitutional disorder, in which, as we have seen, tuberculous disease has its origin, constitutes the most important part of the treatment, as it is during this state and before tuberculous matter is deposited, that curative measures are most effectual. Even when tuberculous deposits have taken place, the constitutional disorder demands our chief consideration. It is only when the local disease has advanced so far as to render the cure hopeless, that the latter and its effects claim our undivided attention.

The treatment of tuberculous cachexia must be regulated according to the predominance of particular symptoms, and the individual constitution. In many cases the most prominent derangement is a disordered state of the digestive organs,—in others a morbid state of the skin : some constitutions present a torpid and inactive condition of the whole system, with a languid circulation and deficient nervous sensibility ; others, characters directly opposite. It is evident, therefore, that although the treatment is to be conducted upon the same general principles, and the same objects are to be attained in all cases, it must be adapted to the varying circumstances of each individual case.

As it rarely happens that the organs and functions more immediately connected with nutrition do not manifest evident derangement, our first and most particular attention must be directed to them : if derangement exists there, we may feel assured that we shall make little progress in improving the general health until it is corrected. Although disorder of the digestive organs in tuberculous persons, no doubt, varies in its characters, there is one prevailing form, already noticed under the name of ' Strumous Dyspepsia,' which I consider of so much importance in a practical point of view, that I shall trespass upon the reader's indulgence by recapitulating some of its leading features. The tongue is generally preternaturally red along the margins and at the extremity, where it also presents numerous small bright red points: the back part is more or less furred according to the duration of the affection. The appetite is generally good, very often craving ;—the bowels, though occasionally loose, are mostly costive; in either case the evacuations are pale, and frequently contain food in an undigested state. The urine is often high-coloured and turbid : the skin is generally dry, although copious perspirations are common, particularly during the night.

These are the more evident indications of the morbid state of the digestive organs, in a very large majority of scrofulous or tuberculous persons, more especially in early life; and I consider them, together with others which have been more fully noticed (Chapter II.), as evidences of irritation and congestion of the chylopoietic viscera; and when such a state exists, our treatment should in the first place be directed to its removal.

The diet must be strictly regulated : it should be mild and free from all stimulating condiments ; the drink should in general be water, or toast or barley water. When there are thirst and a disposition to fever, mild saline medicines will be useful at night: according to my own observation, the best is the common citrate of potass mixture with a small proportion of nitre. Small doses of mercurial chalk, at bed-time, every second or third day, and some gentle aperient medicine on the following morning, will also be generally necessary. In some cases more active purgatives are required. Where there is much torpor of the bowels and defective biliary secretion, it may be necessary to begin with calomel followed by senna, or by rhubarb and magnesia; a combination of rhubarb, carbonate of soda and tartarised soda also answers well as an aperient in cases where there is a congested state of the mucous membrane, with little irritation; and in such cases calomel is often preferable to the milder preparations of mercury. The object being, not to purge much, but to augment and improve the biliary and other secretions of the chylopoietic viscera, and to induce regularity in the alvine evacuations, the alterative and aperient medicines must be modified accordingly. The occasional use of the warm-bath, and daily friction over the whole surface, will also contribute greatly to improve the functions of the skin, and to relieve the irritation and congestion of the internal organs.

Such are the most effectual remedies in the more recent cases of strumous dyspepsia. When the affection is of long standing, the treatment requires to be varied according to the circumstances of individual cases. The mineral acids, sometimes without and at others with light bitters, the taraxacum, sarsaparilla, and mineral waters, may all be required in their turn.

When the tongue becomes clean, and the alvine evacuations natural and regular, medicines which act on the constitution generally may be adopted with every prospect of benefit. But until the disorder of the digestive organs is removed, or greatly abated, all such medicines will prove prejudicial, or at best but of temporary advantage. While it is present, steel, bark, and other tonics, and wine and a stimulating diet, are most injurious; yet, from scrofula being erroneously considered to arise from pure debility, such are the remedies and the regimen very generally prescribed for scrofulous children,—with how little success I appeal to the experience of the profession to decide.

Before I leave this subject, I would earnestly call the attention of the profession to the pathological state of the digestive organs which has been pointed out. It constitutes one of the most constant features of the tuberculous constitution; and when it is more generally understood, the treatment of strumous diseases will become comparatively simple, and be attended with corresponding success. I do not hesitate to say, that although the tonic treatment at present adopted may give a temporary degree of strength and tone to the system, it very generally tends to augment and confirm the evil which it is intended to remove. I would not be

understood to condemn tonic remedies, more especially chalybeates: on the contrary, I acknowledge
their great utility, but I must object to their un-
timely employment: before they can prove of permanent benefit, the irritation of the gastric system
must be removed or greatly abated, and the functions of the whole chylopoietic viscera in a normal
state. This object being effected, tonics, internal
and external, change of air, and such other means
as act by exciting and bracing the general system,
will prove of great utility.

Having premised these remarks on the most important pathological condition connected with tuberculous diseases, I shall now proceed to notice
the various medicines which are most useful in correcting the cachectic state of the system which precedes and accompanies the formation of tubercles.

The remedies which appear most deserving of
attention with this view are mercury, iodine, antimony, sulphur, taraxacum, sarsaparilla, mineral
waters, alkalies, lime-water, the muriates of lime
and of barytes, and chalybeates.

ALTERATIVES.

MERCURY.—The influence of this medicine on
the secreting functions of the liver renders it a very
valuable remedy in the tuberculous constitution;
but as it seldom fails to prove injurious when
carried beyond its alterative effect on the hepatic

system, its use requires great caution, especially in irritable nervous temperaments.

Of all the preparations of mercury, calomel is the most efficient: there are few remedies more valuable—none, in my opinion, more abused. In a congestive state of the hepatic system, it is highly useful; but when the mucous surface of the alimentary canal is in an irritable condition, it must be employed with care. The injudicious manner in which children are dosed with calomel and drenched with black draughts is the destruction of many. Against this pernicious system of treatment I would enter my strongest protest.

Calomel, when given in doses suited to the patient's age and to the state of the digestive organs, repeated only at considerable intervals, and followed by mild aperients, forms a valuable remedy in many cases of tuberculous cachexia, more especially in torpid constitutions. When it is necessary to continue the action of mercury on the liver for any time, after a few doses of calomel, I generally give the preference to the milder preparations, such as the hydrargyrum cum cretâ: this, or the blue-pill, given in such doses and at such intervals as shall prevent its producing irritation of the mucous surfaces of the alimentary canal, and followed by some gentle laxative, is very useful in cases where an imperfect biliary secretion and a torpid state of the bowels are prominent symptoms.

Mercury is usually, and I think very properly, prescribed in combination with some narcotic, such as hyoscyamus or conium. The utmost circumspection on the part of the practitioner is necessary in the administration of mercury in strumous constitutions, especially in the case of children. It should be alternated with purgatives, and laid aside as soon as the object for which it was given is attained. Such, at least, is the result of my observation of the effects of this powerful medicine.

IODINE.—The action of iodine on the animal economy in a great degree resembles that of mercury. They both promote the excretory functions, and it is thus, most probably, that they increase the activity of the assimilative functions. Mercury is more quick in its operation than iodine, and we are better acquainted with its management; but the operation of iodine on the economy appears to be more general. Its action on the uterine system is decided; on the secreting functions of the liver and kidneys its operation is also evident; and it appears to promote the insensible perspiration. It thus diminishes abdominal plethora, promoting the activity of the eliminative functions, and, through them, of the assimilative. But in whatever way we may attempt to explain its mode of operation, the beneficial effects of iodine on stru-

mous constitutions are undoubted. Under its influence, when it is judiciously employed, the
patient recovers flesh, strength, and colour: hitherto pale, relaxed, and feeble, he becomes full,
strong, and florid ; glandular swellings disappear
or are greatly reduced; scrofulous ulcers heal ;
swellings of the joints are reduced, and the limbs
restored to their natural proportions ; and the condition of the whole animal economy is greatly
improved.*

As with all other medicines exerting a powerful
action on the system, the employment of iodine
requires judgment. When the digestive organs
are in a state of irritation, or when an inflammatory state of the mucous membrane prevails,
it should not be given ; in great irritability and
sensibility of the nervous system it is scarcely admissible ; and when there is much emaciation, it
is a very doubtful remedy.

With these exceptions iodine or its salts may often
be employed with advantage, I believe, in the treatment of tuberculous cachexia, and in many of the
local diseases arising out of this condition. In congestion of the glandular and cellular system, and in
cutaneous affections of a strumous character, the effects of iodine are often remarkable. Dr. Todd lately

---

* Baudelocque, op. citat.

cured a very severe and obstinate case of *favus,*
one of the scrofulous eruptions, with iodine alone.
In almost all forms of tuberculous disease affecting
the external parts, when the state of the digestive
organs or nervous system of the patient does not
contra-indicate it, iodine may be used with advantage. Its effects on tuberculous disease of the
internal organs will be better considered further
on; my object at present being to point out its value
as a remedy in correcting tuberculous cachexia.
The beneficial effects of iodine are most remarkable
in childhood and youth; and it is at this age that
its aid is most required.

M. Baudelocque's method of using iodine, and
the preparations employed by him, appear to me
judicious; and the success which attended his administration of it in the Children's Hospital at
Paris, which is not the most favourable situation
for scrofulous patients, proves that the practice
was well directed. M. Baudelocque gave iodine
and the hydriodate of potash dissolved together
in water. His proportions were one-eighth of
a grain of iodine, and one-fourth. of a grain of
hydriodate of potash to an ounce of water. When
the solution was stronger than this, it irritated
the stomach and induced vomiting. He gradually
increased the dose of this solution from one
ounce to twelve ounces twice a day—that is, to
six grains of the hydriodate of potash, and three

grains of the iodine daily : he never increased the dose beyond this. After having continued the iodine in the dose which he judged to be adapted to each case, for from three to six weeks, he laid it aside for several weeks, during which he put the patient on the use of diluents, and gave one or two saline purgatives. In this way he often continued the medicine for many months, and generally with the effect of improving the general health and embonpoint of the young patients in a remarkable degree. M. Baudelocque attributes, and I think justly, the good effects which he so generally obtained from the iodine to his careful mode of using it.

In some cases the iodine produced cardialgia, which was relieved by combining with it a vinous tincture of bark, as recommended by Coindet. In one instance only did it produce marasmus. In some cases the mouth became ulcerated, the ulcers having the same odour as that arising from mercurial sores.

In girls he found it often necessary to lay aside the iodine, in consequence of their suffering from severe headach about the period of the catamenia. Such headachs never occurred in boys. With the internal use of iodine, Dr. Baudelocque combined its external application in the form of bath, with some advantage. He also found friction with ioduretted ointments useful in promoting the reduction

of glandular swellings, and the effect was increased
by occasionally changing the form of ointment.*

The method of M. Baudelocque appears to me to
admit of improvement, at least in many cases, by
a more frequent use of purgative medicines, where
the state of the patient required these. Respecting
the particular condition of the patients submitted
to the action of iodine, and its direct or more obvious effects, M. Baudelocque's work, and indeed
almost all other works on the subject, with which
I am acquainted, are very defective in the necessary information. Yet the more immediate and
evident effects of medicines deserve our best attention : this is a kind of knowledge much neglected,
and yet is essential, as enabling us to direct the application of medicines to particular cases. M. Baudelocque's practice of intermitting the use of the

* The following are the ointments employed by M. Baudelocque:—

> R Iodinæ, gr. xii.
> Hydriodat. Potassæ, ʒi.
> Adipis, ʒi.   M.

> R Iodid. Plumbi, ʒi.
> Adipis, ʒi.   M.

> R Prot-Iodid. Hydrargyri, gr. xxx.
> Adipis, ʒi.   M.

The first and last ointments, he observes, produce in some
cases a sensation of heat, of pricking, or of burning, which may
continue a quarter of an hour.

iodine from time to time, and watching its effects on the system, I consider highly judicious. It would be still better to make the periods of suspension at shorter intervals.

Before iodine is prescribed, the digestive organs should be free from irritation and congestion. The use of mercury may frequently precede that of iodine with great advantage. The powerful and decided effect of the former in promoting the biliary secretion and unloading the intestines, will prepare the system for the more slow and general operation of the iodine. The employment of this medicine does not supersede the general regimen and mode of treatment of tuberculous cachexia; nor does this interfere with the operation of iodine.

For further details on the use of iodine, I beg to refer to the late excellent work of Baudelocque on the subject; to the memoirs of Coindet, of De Carro, of Brera, and of Lugol, among foreign authors; and to the writings of Baron, of Gardiner, of Mansel, and of Bardsley in this country. I would also recommend the perusal of Dr. Jahn's memoir on the injurious effects of iodine when injudiciously prescribed.*

ANTIMONY.—This medicine has been much extolled for its alterative powers. The once-cele-

* De la Maladie Iodique, ou des Désordres qu'entraine à sa suite l'emploi trop long temps continué de l'Iode.—*Journal Complémentaire*, tom. xxxv.

brated anti-hectic of Poterius consisted of oxide of antimony and tin. Hufeland expresses the highest opinion of antimony in correcting the strumous diathesis.* I have not often administered its preparations alone as alteratives, but very frequently in combination with other medicines of the same class. When a disposition to fever, with a dry hot skin, or bronchial irritation, exists, I consider antimony a valuable addition to any mild alterative which may be suited to the case; but it must be given with caution, on account of its depressing effects. As an emetic, the tartarized antimony is considered superior to every other in emulging the biliary system.

TARAXACUM.—I consider taraxacum a very valuable medicine in tuberculous constitutions, from its power of diminishing abdominal plethora, and its especial influence on the urinary and biliary secretions. Hufeland strongly recommends it every spring in the treatment of scrofula, and the translator of his work regards it as an efficacious remedy in the mesenteric disease of infants, and in the congestions of the abdominal viscera which are the consequences of intermittent fevers; he also cites Zimmermann's opinion that it is the best remedy for the dispersion of pulmonary tubercles.†

* Op. cit. p. 166.   † Id. p. 275.

Kaempf and his followers made extensive use of taraxacum in the form of enemata in almost all the chronic diseases of the abdomen, and, if we may judge from the reputation which their method of treatment acquired, with great success.*

After a few doses of mercurial alteratives, a course of taraxacum, steadily pursued for several weeks during the spring or summer, will often produce a very beneficial effect. The freshly expressed juice is the form in which it is usually given on the continent, where it is considered infinitely superior to every other preparation of the plant, and I think that it deserves a preference when it can be procured. The extract, however, when well prepared, contains, I believe, the virtues of the plant.† I usually prescribe it in combination

---

* See chap. on PATHOLOGY, p. 262.

† There is a marked difference in the appearance of the extracts of this plant in the shops, and, there is reason to believe, not less difference in their medical qualities. The extract is generally prepared in the spring, when the root contains little more than a colourless watery fluid. In the autumn the root is charged with a white milky juice, which appears to contain all the virtue of the plant. I would strongly recommend the attention of pharmaceutical chemists to this circumstance. Mr. Houlton's directions for preparing this extract are the best I have seen, and his extract appears superior to every other; still I believe his mode of preparation admits of improvement. See Burnett's Medical Botany, vol. i.

with some tincture of hops and aromatic water,
and in this form find no difficulty in getting
children to take it for weeks. The bowels require
attention, and during its use an occasional laxative
will be beneficial in all cases.

SARSAPARILLA.—Although the powers of sarsaparilla have been very differently estimated, and the
circumstances in which it is most beneficial are by
no means well ascertained, it has long been used as
an alterative. Its influence appears to be chiefly
exerted on the skin; it is, therefore, in cases in
which there is a defective state of the cutaneous
secretion that it promises to be useful. After the
employment of mercurial or other aperient alteratives, a course of sarsaparilla, with warm bathing,
will often prove beneficial. Sarsaparilla is given
also in combination with alkaline medicines.

ALKALIS. — Alkalis have been employed as
alteratives in the treatment of scrofulous diseases,
chiefly with the view of correcting the constitutional diathesis. The theory which gave rise to
their employment, viz. that acidity is the chief
cause of scrofula, is now exploded; still they are
held in considerable repute and are unquestionably
often useful.

The fixed alkalis are mostly employed in this
country, the liquor potassæ, the carbonates of
potash and of soda, being the forms in which they
are chiefly used. Their mode of action is not well

understood; they evidently increase the urinary, and appear to promote the bilious secretion, and to render that of the mucous membranes more fluid. Their alterative action on the skin is also evinced by their abating cutaneous irritation : the effects of the liquor potassæ in correcting the disposition to boils is very remarkable. But, in whatever way they operate, they are certainly beneficial in many tuberculous affections; they also form valuable adjuncts to purgative medicines.

Lime-water has been long held in estimation : Morton prescribed it in combination with the decoction of sarsaparilla; Hufeland, also, speaks in high terms of its efficacy in glandular swellings, in mesenteric disease, and even in incipient tuberculous phthisis.

The Muriates of Lime and of Barytes likewise were, at one time, in great repute in the treatment of scrofulous diseases, and are still held in estimation on the continent. Hufeland considers muriate of barytes equal to mercury and antimony in scrofulous affections of the glands and skin, and Baumes expresses an equally high opinion of it.

During the use of all these alteratives, the warm bath will be productive of considerable benefit. By promoting a free circulation in the cutaneous vessels, it favours the operation of those medicines which act specifically on the surface, relieves internal congestion, and thereby indirectly aids also the action of those alterative remedies which exert their influence on the abdominal secretions.

MINERAL WATERS.

Nature has supplied us with a most valuable class of remedies in mineral waters : when judiciously prescribed, I consider them capable of effecting more benefit than any other class of alterative medicines. But their employment need not interfere with, and does not prevent, the use of other alteratives; on the contrary, as has been already stated, the previous use of the latter often renders the former more efficient.

The operation of mineral waters may be so directed as to promote almost all the secretions and excretions, to influence the functions of almost every organ, and to improve the condition of the whole system. In strumous habits, affected with great abdominal plethora, a defective biliary secretion, and an unhealthy state of the skin, no remedy with which I am acquainted is so well calculated to produce a full alterative effect on the constitution as a well-directed course of alterative and aperient mineral waters, combined with warm bathing. They are not, however, suited to every person of the strumous constitution. In the class of cases just alluded to, their utility is at once apparent; but in young persons of an excitable temperament, the operation of the mildest kind

will scarcely be borne. The waters of this class
in which I have the greatest confidence, and from
which I have observed the most marked benefit, are
those of Ems, of Carlsbad, of Marienbad, and of
Eger. The saline waters of this country, also, such
as those of Cheltenham and Leamington, no doubt
prove useful in many cases.

SULPHUREOUS WATERS.—I consider the mineral
waters of this class the best form of administering
sulphur. Bathing should generally be combined
with their internal use ; and when the water does
not act on the bowels, they should be kept open
by laxatives. Bordeu combined mercurial frictions
with the sulphureous waters of Barège; but this,
I believe, is unnecessary when the patient has been
properly prepared for the operation of the waters
by a course of mercurial or vegetable alteratives,
which, if not always requisite, will very generally
be useful, and render sulphureous and other mineral
waters also more effectual.

Of the warm sulphureous waters, those of the
Pyrenees and of Aix-la-Chapelle are the best on
the continent. In this country we have some excellent cold sulphureous waters, such as those of
Harrowgate, of Croft, &c., in the north of England, and Strathpeffer and Moffat in Scotland.

CHALYBEATE WATERS.—The purer chalybeate
waters have been esteemed valuable remedies in correcting the scrofulous constitution. Morton consi-

dered them the most useful of all preventives of phthisis, and he states that he has seen cases of evident consumption perfectly cured by their use.*

In passing from the subject of mineral waters, I cannot but express my belief that when their powerful effects in the extensive class of diseases which have their origin in abdominal plethora and deficient excretion, together with the mode of exhibiting them, are better understood, they will be more fully appreciated and more generally employed.†

EVACUANTS.

PURGATIVES.—Aperient medicines are chiefly useful in obviating constipation, or in promoting the operation of alteratives; but their employment in tuberculous subjects must be regulated by certain restrictions. In a torpid state of the bowels, with little disposition to irritation of the alimentary canal, active purgatives may be occasionally useful; but I must protest against the indiscriminate practice of strong and often repeated purging which still too generally prevails in the cases under con-

---

* Op. citat. lib. ii. cap. ii. et ix. lib. iii. cap. v.

† I beg to call the attention of my readers to the artificial mineral waters prepared at Brighton, which supply an accurate imitation of the most esteemed waters of Germany. At this well-conducted establishment an opportunity is also afforded of varying the water according to the state of the patient, the advantages of which are obvious.

sideration. It is lamentable to observe the
injurious effects of this practice in the debility
which it produces, and in the permanent irritation
which it often establishes in the digestive organs.
Although I consider that abdominal congestion forms
a most important part in the pathology of tuberculous diseases, I regard the frequent repetition of
harsh purgatives as the worst possible means of
remedying it : a few doses of active aperient medicine often give relief, by the copious discharge
which is excited from the liver and mucous surfaces;
but the frequent repetition of this operation rarely
fails to do injury. Entertaining these views, I read
with much pleasure the strong opinion of Dr. Stokes
of Dublin, on this subject. Speaking of the influence
of gastro-enteric disease in accelerating the fatal
termination of phthisis, he says, " I feel satisfied,
that under a different mode of treatment from that
ordinarily employed, this complication would be
much less frequently observed ; as in numerous
instances I have known it to be induced clearly by
the use of purgative medicines. If ever there was
a case in which we should be cautious in giving
medicines of this description, it is in incipient or
threatened phthisis, on account of the great liability
that exists to inflammation and ulceration of the
digestive tube; yet, in all those cases, which, in
conformity with the prejudice of the day, are supposed to arise from a *disordered state of the stomach*

—*of the digestive apparatus—a depraved state of
the biliary organs—atony of the chylopoietic viscera,
&c. &c.* a set of terms invented to cloak ignorance,
and conveying no single clear idea to the mind,
this practice is constantly pursued—a diarrhœa is
established, and the digestive apparatus becomes
indeed disordered, more from the remedies than
the disease."*

The prevalent use of calomel and strong purgatives in delicate strumous children is productive of a
degree of mischief which is not sufficiently known:
the great error in administering such medicines is
the excessive doses in which they are so often given,
and their too frequent repetition. Where they are
judiciously given, and their repetition is regulated
according to the nature of the case, especially
when a course of alterative medicine forms a part
of the treatment, they may be made very useful
in the correction of the strumous habit; but in
young delicate persons of a strumous constitution
no class of remedies requires to be exhibited with
more caution.

EMETICS.—In a disorder in which a deranged
state of the first passages forms a prominent symptom, emetics cannot fail to be useful. Hufeland
always begins the treatment of scrofula with emetics,
and continues to repeat them occasionally. Baumes

* Dublin Journal of Med. and Chem. Science, vol. ii. p. 59,
60.

recommends them as indispensable, and observes, correctly I think, that their place cannot be supplied by purgatives. The good effects of emetics in children are often very striking, and they are at present too much neglected. When the upper part of the alimentary canal is loaded, as is indicated by a thickly furred state of the tongue, fetid health and loss of appetite, common symptoms in strumous children, an emetic proves very useful, and may be repeated from time to time in such cases with great advantage.

TONICS.

In a disease in which debility is one of the principal features, it is not surprising that tonics should suggest themselves to the mind both of the medical attendant and the patient.

IRON.—Chalybeates have an excellent effect in some young persons of a tuberculous constitution. In those who have a languid circulation, a soft relaxed state of muscle, and a pale, bloodless appearance, they are superior, I believe, to every other remedy; but the indiscriminate exhibition of them is productive of much mischief. Before benefit can be derived from chalybeates, the digestive organs must be free from irritation; otherwise, however great may be the debility, they will generally do harm. The injudicious manner in which the preparations of iron are too commonly prescribed in all cases of scrofula and debility is productive of more injury than is imagined : although they may give a temporary support to the system, they rarely fail, when incautiously employed, to confirm the functional derangement, which it should be our first object to remove.

BARK.—Bark is the only other tonic which deserves particular notice. In many cases it is highly useful, especially after any discharge which has left much debility; but the remarks which have been made respecting the use of steel apply also to bark. Dr. Fothergill has pointed out the circumstances in which this medicine is most useful.*

BATHING.

COLD BATH.—As a means of giving tone to the system and enabling it to bear the vicissitudes of climate, the cold bath forms a very valuable remedy. I would strongly recommend that it should be used by children and young persons of a scrofulous constitution during the summer, as being one of the best tonics they can employ. For the bath, sea-water is to be preferred when it can be obtained, and the air of the coast materially contributes to the benefit which is generally experienced from a course of sea-bathing. The same cautions apply

* On the Use of the Cortex Peruvianus in Scrofulous Disorders. *Works*, London, 1781.

to the cold bath as to other tonics;—unless the
functions of the internal organs are in a healthy
state, little advantage will be derived from it.
Before prescribing this remedy, therefore, it is
always necessary to ascertain if the digestive functions in particular are well performed; and when
there are indications of abdominal congestion, it
should be removed by such alterative and aperient
remedies as the case requires, and when the skin is
dry and harsh, it will be proper to employ the warm
bath also as a preliminary measure. But notwithstanding all these precautions, we shall find that
some children cannot bear the shock of the cold bath,
and are positively injured by it; hence its effects
must be closely watched. Unless it is succeeded
by a glow, a feeling of increased strength, and a
keen appetite, it ought to be at once abandoned,
and the warm or tepid sea-water bath substituted.

Cold Sponging.—Delicate persons, who cannot
bear the cold plunge or shower-bath, will often
derive great benefit from having the body rapidly
sponged with cold water, succeeded by friction over
the whole surface. This is particularly serviceable
to young children. The practice of daily sponging
the chest with sea-water or salt and water is also
highly useful, and should generally be adopted by
delicate persons throughout the year. It is a powerful tonic, and most effective in diminishing the
susceptibility to the impressions of cold.

While on the subject of cold bathing, I must not omit to notice the beneficial effects of swimming. With this invigorating exercise, the cold bath is doubly serviceable. Swimming, as Locke recommends, ought to form a part of every boy's education.

TEPID BATH.—In very delicate children much more benefit will be derived from the tepid than the cold bath : the former, indeed, is to them what the latter is to the more robust. The powers of warm and tepid bathing in the treatment of scrofulous children are not sufficiently valued. One of the most powerful means of relieving abdominal congestion, improving the functions of the skin, and giving tone and vigour to the whole system, is a course of warm sea-bathing with active friction over the whole surface after each bath ; the temperature of the bath towards the termination of the course being gradually reduced till it becomes tepid. The opinion that warm baths generally relax is erroneous : they are no doubt debilitating when used by some persons of a weak and relaxed constitution, or when continued too long ; but, when appropriately employed, they generally give tone. I have already remarked that warm bathing greatly promotes the action of alterative medicines ; these two remedies, therefore, when possible, should be combined.*

* The excellent article on BATHING, by Dr. Forbes, in the *Cyclopædia of Practical Medicine*, contains the best and most scientific rules for the use of baths with which I am acquainted.

MEDICATED BATHS.—Of Medicated Baths I have had no practical experience: common salt and the carbonate of soda and potash are the only substances which I have used in this way, and from these I have observed good effects. Baths of malt, of bark, of hemlock, and other substances supposed to have specific effects, have been particularly mentioned by foreign authors. Hufeland states that he has seen surprising benefit derived from hemlock baths, repeated daily for weeks, in removing glandular swellings, cicatrizing ulcers, &c.; and he considers bark and other astringents, when employed in this way, much more useful than when administered internally.

TRAVELLING, SAILING, CLIMATE.

These are valuable means of improving the health of persons of a tuberculous constitution; and when no local disorder exists to prevent their beneficial influence, they may be made powerful remedies in correcting the disposition to tuberculous disease. But these measures must be pursued for a long period; a residence for a few months only in the finest climate, or travelling under the most favourable circumstances, cannot be expected to do much in correcting a constitutional disorder which may have existed from birth. Their positive advantages also depend upon their being adapted to the circumstances of the individual case, and upon a strict attention to the necessary regulations respecting regimen, exercise, &c.; for no measures which act on the system generally will prove of much permanent benefit, unless the local derangements which almost invariably exist in the scrofulous constitution are removed before their adoption. It is from a want of due attention to these circumstances, and from an over-confidence in the unaided effects of the measures which have been alluded to, that so little benefit is often derived from them.

When proper regard is paid to all the circumstances of the patient, and the measure is adopted with the necessary precautions, travelling is attended with many advantages. Independently of its physical effects, the change of scene and the constant succession of new objects exert a direct and most benefical influence on the mental constitution; the mind is engaged, the nervous system is soothed, and a just harmony between the various functions of the economy is established. If the traveller is fond of natural scenery, or takes delight in the practical pursuit of any branch of natural history, the beneficial effects of a residence in a mild climate may be much augmented. For this reason a taste for botany, geology, and similar pursuits, which necessarily imply exercise in the open air, should always be encouraged in young persons of a delicate constitution; the study of marine botany and of the various branches of zoology which can only be pursued on the sea-shore, also contributes greatly, when used with proper precautions, to the amendment of the health.

When more distant journeys or voyages cannot be undertaken, short and repeated voyages and excursions, within the limits of our own country, and on the surrounding seas, during the continuance of mild weather, may be productive of benefit. It is chiefly with the view of avoiding the winter season that foreign residence is recommended; but this subject will be more fully considered when treating of the effects of climate in incipient consumption.

CHAPTER XIV.

THE present chapter is devoted to the consideration of those remedies which have been found most beneficial in the treatment of tuberculous disease of the lungs, or pulmonary consumption properly so called. But in our treatment of local tuberculous disease, the means of correcting tuberculous cachexia, and the functional derangements which usually accompany it, must never be lost sight of.

SECT. I.—GENERAL REMEDIES.

It would be unprofitable to pass under our review all the remedies which have at various times been extolled as capable of curing consumption. The greater number of them were put forth by empirics; and although they acquired some notoriety in their day from popular credulity, it is needless to observe that they have been and ever will be found wholly inadequate to answer the un-

worthy professions held out by the ignorant and
designing pretenders who introduced them. Passing over, therefore, a long list of nostrums which
have been justly banished from rational practice, I
shall merely notice those remedies the beneficial
effects of which are tolerably well established on
the evidence of experience, either in the treatment
of the disease generally, or in the relief of particular symptoms.

BLOODLETTING.

Small and frequently-repeated bleedings have
been recommended by various authors as a means
of curing incipient consumption. Morton employed
bleeding in the early stages of the disease, and for
the prevention of hemoptysis, to the extent of from
six to ten ounces, and, when its repetition was indicated, recurred to it two or three times at proper
intervals. If employed in due season, and aided
by the judicious exhibition of other necessary remedies, he considers it very successful in guarding
against inflammation, congestion, and subsequent
ulceration of the lungs, but positively destructive in
the confirmed stage of phthisis.* But the practice
of repeated bleedings in consumption was first
brought into general notice in this country by
Dovar, whose extravagant partiality for, and ex-

* Op. cit. lib. ii. ch. ii.

cessive employment of, the remedy, probably led to its unmerited disuse. His plan was to bleed to the amount of six or eight ounces every day for the first fortnight, and gradually to increase the period between each repetition of the measure, by employing it at the respective intervals of every second, third, and fifth day for the three successive fortnights.* Mead speaks strongly in favour of frequent bleedings, even when the disease is advanced:—" I have seen cases," he says, " judged almost desperate, where this method of practice succeeded well."† Sir John Pringle says, " In the first stage of a consumption, when the patient complains of pains in his side, constriction at the breast, or hot and restless nights, I have trusted most to small and repeated bleedings: the quantity of blood drawn was from four to seven or eight ounces, once in eight or ten days; and sometimes a vein was opened after shorter intervals."‡ Dr. Monro states that the plan of " taking away from four to eight ounces of blood, whenever the pain of the breast was troublesome, or the patient was hot and restless at nights from the hectic fever, gave the greatest relief of any thing we tried; and

---

* The Ancient Physician's Legacy to his Country. By Thomas Dovar, M.D., p. 26. Lond. 1733.

† Monita et Præcepta Med. c. i. s. x.

‡ Observations on the Diseases of the Army, part iii. ch. iii.

these repeated small bleedings were so far from wasting the patient's strength that they rather seemed to prevent its being exhausted so fast as otherwise it would have been, by allaying the force of the hectic fever."* We must bear in mind that Pringle and Monro were army-physicians, and that their patients were of a class more likely to require and derive advantage from bleeding than the generality of consumptive patients in private life. Fothergill always found benefit from repeated venesection, except in delicate constitutions; and Stoll considered it one of the best remedies that could be employed in phthisis connected with hemoptysis. More recently several physicians have spoken favourably of the practice of bloodletting. Dr. Hosack of New York states that he has " in many instances employed it with the most happy effect in incipient phthisis, even when strong hereditary predisposition existed."† Dr. Cheyne of Dublin has also given a very favourable opinion of this practice in hemoptysis, and in incipient pulmonary consumption; in both of which he states that " small bleedings may be practised with safety, and often, if I mistake not, with more advantage than any other remedy in use."‡ Dr. Cheyne's

* Account of the Diseases in the British Military Hospitals in Germany, &c. p. 131.

† American Med. and Philos. Register, vol. ii. p. 470.

‡ Dublin Hospital Reports, vol. v.

view in adopting this practice is to subdue the inflammatory state of the lungs produced by the irritation of tubercles, and to arrest the progress of
the disease in its early stage : he employed small
bleedings once every week or ten days in cases
which he conceived to be incipient phthisis, " and
with a degree of success which forbids the relin-
quishment of the practice."

The greater number of the advocates of this
practice evidently adopted it, not only after tuberculous disease of the lungs had taken place, but
after it had become complicated with inflammation.
But the utility of bloodletting is not limited to this
stage of the disease ; before the existence of tuberculous disease of the lungs, it may often be employed with advantage to remove pulmonary congestion. When this exists, a moderate bleeding
will always, I believe, be useful; and when employed as soon as the congestion is evident, it may
prevent hemorrhage or inflammation, and perhaps
the deposition of tuberculous matter. When the
patient has been subject to natural discharges of
blood from the nose, or otherwise, venesection is
the more likely to prove beneficial. It rarely happens, I believe, that general bleeding requires to
be frequently repeated, if the patient be put upon
a proper regimen, and the necessary remedies are
employed to diminish pulmonary and abdominal
plethora. When the practice of frequent bleedings

is adopted, the quantity of blood abstracted should be less each time, and the intervals increased.

The employment of general bloodletting, and even the local abstraction of blood, in consumption, requires, in my opinion, great judgment and circumspection. The more general error is the abstraction of too great a quantity of blood at a time ; treating the disease as if it were a purely inflammatory one, and forgetting that the inflammatory symptoms are merely consecutive upon tubercles, and that the constitution of the consumptive patient is little capable of replacing the blood too often lavishly drawn. But keeping clearly before us the condition of our patient, the nature of his constitution, and the pathological condition of the lungs, and considering that the utmost benefit which we can generally expect or derive from the practice, is the removal or diminution of congestion or inflammation, complicated with and often dependent on the presence of tubercles;—keeping all these circumstances in view, blood may be abstracted with advantage at any stage of consumption, when the symptoms require it. " In the present state of our knowledge," observes Dr. Carswell, " there is, perhaps, no practical rule regarding the local treatment of tuberculous affections of equal importance with that which is founded on the pathological fact of inflammation being the frequent, if not the necessary consequence of the mere mechanical pre-

sence of the material by means of which we recognize the local existence of these affections. To
protect the individual and the affected organ from
the influence of all those agents, internal and external, which tend to create an inordinate degree
of excitement, or favour the development of active
congestion or inflammation, is the rule to which
we allude, and to which there can be no exception
in the treatment of tuberculous diseases." After
pulmonary congestion has been diminished by general bleeding, the abstraction of blood by means
of cupping or leeches, when further depletion is
necessary, has a very beneficial effect.

EMETICS.

From an early period in the history of medicine,
emetics have been employed in the treatment of
consumption; and, although they were prescribed
with various views by different practitioners, their
beneficial effects, when judiciously exhibited, have
been generally acknowledged. Some considered
them chiefly useful in unloading the stomach and
biliary system; some used them as the means of
suppressing pulmonary hemorrhage and inflammation; while others, without attempting to explain
their mode of operation, regarded them as capable of curing consumption in its early stages. It
is my present purpose to examine the grounds upon
which this last opinion rests, and the circumstances

under which emetics may be exhibited with the
greatest prospect of advantage.

We have the positive testimony of several practical physicians in favour of the remarkable benefit
derived from gentle emetics repeated at short
intervals during the early stages of tuberculous
phthisis. Morton states that after bleeding they
are of great utility in the cure of this disease, and
that they will often check it in its early stages.
The opinion of this eminent and sagacious physician is so clearly and strongly expressed that I
shall give it in his own words: " A quâ vomitione
non tantùm ventriculus humorum saburrâ oppressus
relevari, et nausea inde nata tolli, et digestio res-
titui possint, (quæ omnia non sunt flocci habenda,)
verùm etiam moles humorum jam pulmonibus im-
pactorum, harum partium exagitatione inter vomen-
dum, insignitèr expectorari solet, unà cum notabili
relevatione ponderis gravativi à mole istâ effecti.
Atque hoc ritu non tantùm *plurimos empiricos* vidi,
cum successu felici, sese omnem incipientem phthi-
sin curaturos gloriari, verùm etiam ipse ego ratione
et experientiâ fretus sæpissimè phthiseos incipi-
entis progressum, eodem modo, brevi temporis
spatio, præpedivi."* Again, in regard to cases
complicated with hysteria and hypochondriasis, he
says, " vomitoria verò lenia, et ægri viribus æqua-

* Op. cit. lib. ii. cap. viii.

lia, opitulando cerebro et nervis, in principio morbi, instar miraculi hujusmodi phthisicos relevare solent."* Since Morton's time, emetics have been recommended by several eminent physicians; Dr. Simmons warmly advocates the practice, and lays down some excellent directions for their employment.† Dr. Parr says that " no remedy is so generally useful as a slight emetic frequently repeated; and could phthisis be ever cured, it would be by the joint action of emetics and blisters."‡ Dr. Bryan Robinson,§ Dr. Thomas Reid,‖ and Dr. Marryat,¶ have each urged the employment of emetics in still more forcible language, firmly convinced, by their own experience, of the value of the remedy in the early stages of phthisis. Dr. Dumas of Montpellier, one of the translators of Dr. Reid's work, also supports the practice; and, more recently, Bayle, a high authority, has mentioned emetics, frequently repeated, among the most valuable remedies in the early stages of phthisis. The late Dr. Young, whose

* Op. cit. lib. iii. cap. iv.

† Practical Observations on the Treatment of Consumption, p. 67.

‡ Lond. Med. Dict., art. *Emetics.*

§ Observations on the Virtues and Operations of Medicines, 1752, p. 146, et seq.

‖ Essay on the Nature and Cure of the Phthisis Pulmonalis, 1782.

¶ Therapeutics, or the Art of Healing, 1817, p. 45.

extensive researches on the literature of phthisis are well known, observes, " It is remarkable that a very great majority of the cures of consumption, which are related by different authors, have either been performed by emetics, or by decidedly nauseating remedies."[*]

The most recent and extensive experiments with emetics are those by Dr. Giovanni de Vittis, chief physician to the military hospitals of the Neapolitan army. In the military hospital at Capua, where the greater number of phthisical patients of the army are sent, antimonial emetics were tried in every case. From the 1st of May 1828, to the 18th of January 1832, there were sent out of the hospital perfectly cured, " *perfettamente guariti,*" forty cases of *chronic catarrh*, forty-seven of *phthisis* in the first stage, one hundred and two in the second, and twenty-seven in the third, making a total of two hundred and sixteen cures, one hundred and seventy-six of which were cases of phthisis. The mode of treatment consisted in giving, every morning and evening, a tablespoonful of a solution containing three grains of tartarized antimony in five ounces of infusion of elder-flowers, and one ounce of syrup. A second spoonful of the emetic mixture was given at the end of a quarter of an hour when the first dose did not produce vomiting. The

---

[*] Practical and Historical Treatise on Consumptive Diseases.

patients were at the same time put upon a light farinaceous diet, composed chiefly of rice, chocolate, and biscuits.* If the antimony excited brisk purging, it was omitted for some days, and roasted ipecacuan and digitalis, which are said to produce wonderful effects in curing this diarrhœa, were administered in doses of a grain of each, and repeated every hour or oftener, until the diarrhœa ceased.

Although we may be permitted to question the permanency of all the cures, especially of those in the advanced stage, we cannot doubt that the practice must generally have produced very beneficial effects.

The extent to which vomiting was carried by the advocates of the practice, may well surprise the practitioners of the present day; Reid says that an emetic may be taken every morning and evening with perfect safety for months; Richter gives the case of a woman, aged forty, who took six hundred emetics in ten years; and Robinson states the case of a consumptive patient, subject to repeated at-

---

* This report is taken from an Italian medical journal, Annali Universali di Medicina, Dicembre, 1832; as I have not yet succeeded in procuring the original work, " Observazioni ed esperienze sulla tisi polmonare seguite da un metodo particolare per la cura di tal malattia; del dottor *Giovanni de Vittis*, primo medico degli Ospedali militari dell'armata di terra di S.M.—Napoli, 1832."

tacks of hemoptysis, who was kept alive for eight years by taking three ipecacuan emetics every week during that period. There can be no doubt that the physicians who employed emetics thus extensively were fully assured of the advantages which they produced, and their patients, we may conclude, must have been equally sensible of the benefit derived from them, otherwise it is scarcely credible that a practice so disagreeable would have been prescribed or persevered in. But if such beneficial effects were obtained from the employment of this remedy, it may well excite surprise that it has been allowed to fall into disuse; for at present emetics are merely used as palliatives to relieve particular symptoms, and are by no means generally considered of importance in the cure of consumption. Two causes may be adduced in explanation of this fact; the first, the disagreeable nature of the remedy; the second, the want of firmness and decision on the part of the physician in enforcing a practice, the value and operation of which he could not satisfactorily comprehend. If I can succeed in removing the latter objection by showing how emetics may prove the efficient means of preventing phthisis, the former difficulty will be easily overcome.

I have already stated, as the result of Dr. Carswell's researches, that tuberculous matter is first deposited on the free surfaces of mucous membranes, in all those organs into the structure of which they enter. In the lungs, the extreme branches of the bronchi and the air-cells form the primary and principal seat of tuberculous matter; from the structure of these parts, also, it is most likely to be retained. To prevent such accumulation and retention is a matter of the greatest importance. Now the power of emetics in augmenting and ejecting the bronchial secretion is well established ; we can conceive, therefore, how the repeated action of emetics may prevent the deposition, or at least the retention, of tuberculous matter in the bronchial ramifications and air-cells, and thus prevent the *localization* of the disease, and give time for the correction of the constitutional disorder. The utility of emetics in cases of threatened consumption may be thus partly explained.

I cheerfully acknowledge that my attention was first particularly directed to the benefit which may be derived from emetics in consumption, by Dr. Carswell's researches into the primary seat of tubercle, and whatever advantages may be hereafter experienced from the adoption of the practice, the merit justly belongs to him. If the researches of this enlightened pathologist had led to no other result than the establishment of the important fact, that tuberculous matter is first and most generally deposited on mucous surfaces, and that it may be expelled from them in the way described, he would have conferred a great benefit on mankind.*

But although I regard the action of emetics on the pulmonary system as one of their most valuable effects, I am not disposed to limit their influence to this, but consider that their determining the circulation to the surface and promoting the biliary secretion constitute very important parts of their operation. They restore the secretions which are usually deficient in the tuberculous constitution, tend to diminish abdominal congestion, and equalize the circulation; hence they may be ranked, as Dr. Reid justly observes, among the most powerful alterative medicines which we possess.

The choice of emetics, the period of employing them, and the frequency with which they may be repeated, are not matters of indifference. Morton preferred and generally prescribed squills; that used by Marryat, and called by him the " dry emetic," consisted of one grain of tartar emetic and

* I am aware that all morbid anatomists are not satisfied of the correctness of Dr. Carswell's views, and that objections have been urged against them in the periodical press and otherwise; but the arguments which have been adduced have little weight with one who knows the minute and patient researches of Dr. Carswell, and the pure spirit of philosophical inquiry which directs them; and I hesitate not to predict that the more thoroughly the subject is investigated, the more fully will the views of this enlightened pathologist be borne out and established.

three of ipecacuan, taken fasting, without drinking any liquids during its operation. When the diarrhœa was severe, his emetic consisted of four grains of ipecacuan and one of sulphate of copper. Dr. Senter prefers this combination of sulphate of copper and ipecacuan; he considers it one of the most safe and efficacious emetics in the Materia Medica.* He gave from seven to ten grains of each in the morning fasting, and, if necessary, increased this dose. Reid preferred gentle doses of ipecacuan, sufficient to cause puking once or twice; and Simmons recommends sulphate of copper as superior to any other. Ipecacuan is, perhaps, the safest emetic for repeated use, although it is uncertain in its operation, I fear often owing to the difference in the quality of the drug. The emetics which act most quickly, such as the sulphate of zinc and sulphate of copper, would be the kind of emetics best suited for consumptive patients. The emetic should be so managed as to produce a very gentle effect, and a small quantity of fluid only should be taken to promote its action. For this purpose, tepid chamomile tea is particularly well suited. When the biliary system is much loaded, an antimonial emetic may be useful in the first instance, as it appears to possess more power

---

* Practical Observations on Phthisis Pulmónalis, by J. Senter, M.D.—*Trans. Coll. Physicians, Philadelphia.*

than other emetics in promoting a free discharge of bile.

Morton thought it best to administer the emetic towards evening, and to repeat it every third or fourth day, three or four times, when the patient could bear it and its repetition was indicated. Simmons, Marryat, and Reid thought the morning the best time; and when it is considered that the bronchial secretions accumulate during sleep, there are certainly good reasons for coinciding in their opinion as a general rule; although circumstances may occur to render evening the proper time for the exhibition of the emetic: if given before going to bed, it may in some cases prevent fever and promote sleep.

Simmons began by administering emetics twice a week until the symptoms were relieved, and then repeated them every second day, or even every day for several days together, with good effects. Marryat gave his dry emetic twice or thrice a week: Reid employed ipecacuan every morning, repeating it occasionally in the evening; and he says that this plan may be continued for several months with perfect safety. The repetition of the emetic must, in my opinion, be regulated according to the nature of the case. When it is given with the view of preventing the deposition of tuberculous matter, it may, perhaps, be sufficient to repeat it once or twice a week. When the case is more urgent, and the patient is threatened with the deposition of tuberculous matter in the lungs, or when its presence is already suspected, emetics may be much more frequently repeated : but in all cases it will be necessary to watch their effects on the gastric system, and to suspend the use of them the moment they appear to excite irritation there. During the intervals between the emetics, ipecacuan, alkalies, and other medicines which have the effect of promoting the bronchial secretion, should be given; and this practice may also be adopted in cases in which emetics are not admissible. One of the most important effects of this practice is an increased secretion from the bronchial membrane. This, in Dr. Carswell's view, is the great object to be aimed at, as the more free and fluid the bronchial secretion is, the less will be the chance of any deposit being retained in the air-cells or extreme bronchial ramifications.

Having said thus much on the subject of emetics and their operation, it is right to state that my own experience of the practice has not yet been very considerable ; but I think I shall be justified in earnestly calling the attention of the profession to it, as holding out the rational hope of being made one of the most efficient means of preventing the localization of tuberculous disease of the lungs in many cases, and perhaps of removing it in some others. For myself, I do not hesitate to say that, resting on the discovery of Dr. Carswell, and on the strong testimony of the respectable writers whose authority I have cited, I shall continue to avail myself of every fair occasion to put the practice to the test of experience. That it is a safe practice, when adopted with discernment, we have abundant proof, even when it is carried to an extent which we deem unnecessary.*

If the observations which have just been made should bring into more general use the employment of gentle emetics in tuberculous cachexia and the early stages of consumption, I trust that the measure will not be adopted without that judgment and circumspection which can alone render any active practice useful, or even safe. To have recourse at once to emetics in every instance of threatened phthisis, without fully inquiring into all the circumstances of the case, would be highly injudicious. We shall find that, although emetics may be freely given in one class of cases, they cannot be safely exhibited in another without preparing the patient

---

* Dr. Witt, physician to the Infirmary of Bedford, has long been in the habit of using emetics extensively in his practice. In answer to my inquiry, if he had found them useful in incipient tuberculous disease of the lungs? he writes, " It has fallen to my lot, in our Infirmary here, for the last seven years to have the management of a multitude of pulmonary cases, and when I have been successful, I have in my own mind attributed that success mainly to the unsparing and persevering use of emetics."

for them by bleeding, purgatives, and other anti-phlogistic measures; and that, in a third class, where gastric irritation is a prominent symptom, they are altogether inadmissible. There is a state of the mucous membranes of the alimentary canal which frequently attends consumption even in its earliest stages, and which I consider as strongly contra-indicating the use of emetics. I have already described this state in a former part of this work, but I may observe that it is attended with the following symptoms:—the internal fauces are red, congested, and swollen, the posterior part of the pharynx is also of a deep red, and often partially dry and shining; the tongue is red, there are generally thirst, and some epigastric tenderness on pressure.

When tuberculous matter is deposited in the lungs to a considerable extent, the period has passed when much benefit is to be expected from emetics, and the case will require much consideration before the employment of them; the abstraction of blood, both generally and locally, and a discharge established over the part by blisters or other means, will be useful and may be even necessary in many cases, before emetics can be safely administered; and when there is a disposition to pulmonary inflammation, small doses of tartarized antimony, and medicines which promote the bronchial secretions, may be employed with benefit, and,

in some cases, will be preferable to actual vomiting.
Alkalis have been considered valuable medicines in
promoting the secretion of the mucous surfaces, and
may, therefore, be advantageously prescribed during
the use of emetics. In short, while recommending a
cautious employment of emetics in the early stages
of consumption, I would not be understood to
advise emetics alone, but merely that they should
constitute a part of the treatment in those cases in
which their exhibition is not contra-indicated. The
other remedial means which are adapted to the
case must be employed at the same time : indeed
it is no small recommendation of the practice of
emetics, that it need not interfere with the general
treatment which may be considered most suitable
to the condition of the patient.

IODINE.—The advantages to be derived from
iodine in the treatment of tuberculous cachexia
have been already pointed out ; and its beneficial
effects in scrofula affecting the external parts led
to the hope that it might prove useful also in consumption.   Dr. Morton gives the strongest testimony of the utility of iodine in consumption, that
I have met with : he states that, having used it
extensively, he is able to express an unequivocal
opinion respecting it.   " In a large number of
instances it has appeared, especially in incipient
consumption, to arrest or suspend the tubercular
secretion, and with it the hectic, marasmus, cough,

dyspnœa, and other urgent symptoms. There are some constitutions in which it does not appear to produce any obvious effects, either for better or worse; but in a majority of cases, even in the second stage of phthisis, I have been much gratified with the results. Thus it often relieves the dyspnœa, improves the complexion, and restores the appetite, even when the advanced progress of the disease precludes all hope of recovery. In some instances it has so obviously improved the nutritive function, that patients have increased in flesh by its use, and at the same time recovered, in a considerable degree, a naturally florid complexion."* Dr. Morton is physician to a public hospital, and seems to have had considerable experience. He prescribes the iodine in the form of a solution containing three grains of iodine, and six grains of hydriodate of potash in an ounce of distilled water; from three to five drops of this solution are given morning, noon, and night.

The success of the experiments made with iodine in this country does not by any means correspond with that of Dr. Morton. The result of Dr. Bardsley's observations is very different; after stating the good effects of this medicine in scrofula, he remarks, " It has been my aim to establish the

---

* Illustrations of Pulmonary Consumption, by J. D. Morton, M.D. Philadelphia, 1834.

real virtues of iodine in a tuberculous state of the lungs. In fifteen well-marked examples of incipient phthisis, I employed this medicine with a strict attention to its effects. In five instances, it appeared at first to arrest the further progress of the disease, but the amendment was only temporary, for the tubercles passed slowly but progressively through their several stages, and death was the consequence of the extensive disorganization which occurred in the lungs."* Dr. Baron was, I believe, the first English physician who employed iodine in consumption; he found it produce good effects.† Since the publication of his Illustrations, Dr. Baron has given some striking cases of the removal of tuberculous disease of the abdomen by frictions with iodine in the form of ointment. To his remarks on these cases he adds, " I have reason for believing that tuberculous diseases of the lungs, in their incipient stages, have been removed by treatment corresponding in principle with that just mentioned."‡ Dr. Baron has also favoured me with the two following cases, which were communicated to him by Mr. Cooper, a respectable surgeon of Staunton. The first case was that of a young man who had

* Hospital Facts and Observations, p. 123.

† Illustrations of the Inquiry respecting Tuberculous Diseases, 1822, chap. vi.

‡ Notes on the Use of Iodine, Midland Med. and Surg. Reporter, vol. i. p. 241. 1828-9.

lost his father, and three brothers and three sisters, between the ages of eighteen and twenty-seven, by consumption. Mr. Cooper attended two of them; one he examined after death, and found the greater part of the lungs tuberculous. The last son of the family, the subject of the present notice, walked to Mr. Cooper, the distance of a mile, with great difficulty. He then had cough, pain of left side, difficult breathing, had lost flesh and strength, had night-perspirations, and could not sleep on either side; his pulse was 110. Mr. Cooper considered the case one of well-marked pulmonary consumption. In this state he commenced the hydriodate of potash in solution, the dose being very gradually increased. At the end of three months the improvement in the patient's health was remarkable, and at the end of eight months more he was able to follow his trade, that of a carpenter. Since this period (1825) he has continued well, and is now thirty-two years old, strong and healthy. The impression which this case made in the neighbourhood induced another patient, who had lost his mother, one brother, and two sisters by consumption, to apply to Mr. Cooper. This patient took the solution of hydriodate of potash for two months with little or no advantage; the medicine was continued, and at the end of two months more he improved rapidly: his cough was greatly abated, the pain of his chest ceased, he could run, and ride with ease, and gained flesh.

He has had hemoptysis twice since, which reduced him greatly. The last attack occurred four years ago; since that time he has continued well, has attended to a large estate, and is a keen fox-hunter; is now thirty-five years old, and enjoys good health. He and his father are the only members of his family alive.*

These cases are very interesting, and afford the strongest testimony in favour of iodine in consumption which I have met with. In the very early stage of pulmonary tubercle, when the morbid deposit is limited, it is probable that iodine and its salts may prove very useful.

DIGITALIS.—There is not, perhaps, a medicine in the Materia Medica, concerning the virtues of which inconsumption, medical writers have differed so much as respecting digitalis; some regarding it as possessed of powers beyond all other remedies, others considering it to have very little efficacy; while a third class have even condemned it as pernicious. No better instance of the difficulty of estimating the effects of a medicine can, perhaps, be adduced than the history of digitalis. We find Dr. Beddoes affirming that, in general, when he had all possible evidence of the existence of tubercles, the exhibition of digitalis has been perfectly successful:—" If I specify," he adds,

* Mr. Cooper's communication to Dr. Baron is dated October 25, 1834.

" that it has succeeded in three such cases out of five, I believe I much under-rate the proportion of favourable events."* Now it is not to be credited that Dr. Beddoes would have spoken of digitalis in such terms, unless he had observed some very remarkable effects produced by it. At present we may be permitted to doubt his having all possible evidence of the existence of tuberculous disease of the lungs in many of his cases ; yet making due allowance for this, and for his warm imagination and sanguine character of mind, we cannot doubt that he experienced very beneficial effects from this medicine.

Like several other remedies that have been loudly proclaimed as almost specifics in certain diseases, digitalis has failed, in the hands of others, to maintain the character with which it was introduced to notice by Drake, Beddoes, &c. ; and we would require a series of careful observations to enable us to ascertain its real virtues. In consumption it is now employed chiefly with the view of reducing increased action of the heart, and thereby abating inflammation of the lungs, hemoptysis, and general excitement of the system.

Digitalis is evidently a medicine of great power, although we are not yet acquainted with the peculiar circumstances under which it may be

---

* Essay on Consumption, p. 118.

employed with the greatest advantage in consumption. Of its powers in hemoptysis there can be little doubt: it also possesses considerable efficacy in abating febrile excitement and excitability of the nervous system, and in regulating the action of the heart; hence, when consumption is complicated with disease of this organ, it is a medicine of great utility.

SECT. II.—LOCAL REMEDIES.

The numerous local remedies which have been employed in the treatment of consumption may be considered under two heads;—those applied externally to the thorax, and those applied more directly to the lungs by means of inhalation.

EXTERNAL REMEDIES.—Of the external remedies for preventing or removing congestion and inflammation of the lungs, the abstraction of blood by means of cupping or leeches is one of the most effectual; and there are few cases in which it will not be useful at some period in the course of the disease. In young persons predisposed to consumption, and when pulmonary congestion is present, I consider cupping on the upper parts of the chest very beneficial. A few ounces may be abstracted at intervals, and the good effects of this may be increased by dry-cupping employed at the same time. When tuberculous deposits exist in the lungs, the same practice, judiciously applied, may be the means of preventing or subduing inflammation in the surrounding pulmonary tissue. The application of leeches has been objected to on account of the exposure of the chest which is supposed necessary; but, if the bleeding be properly managed, little risk need be apprehended from this cause. Fomentations or wet cloths are unnecessary: a warm poultice, or dry warm cloths frequently changed, favour the flow of blood more effectually than wet cloths, as has been shown by Dr. Osborne.* The flow of blood may likewise be promoted by covering the leech-bites with cupping-glasses.

I consider cupping on the chest more effectual in general than leeches. Leeches, however, are perhaps equally beneficial in irritation of the bronchial membrane, and preferable when the larynx and trachea are affected, as they may be applied nearer the seat of disease. I would, however, caution the young practitioner against the too free application of leeches in laryngeal irritation in phthisical subjects.

COUNTER-IRRITANTS.—Among the various remedies which have been employed in consumption,

---

* Dublin Med. Journ.

counter-irritants have long occupied a chief place.
They differ considerably in their effects : some, as
the common rubefacients, produce a temporary irritation only, without any discharge; others, as can-
tharides, excite a copious serous discharge; and
others, as tartar emetic, produce deep pustular
eruptions; while setons and issues cause a more
permanent puriform discharge from the subcutaneous tissue. All these applications are useful,
and each is applicable to particular circumstances.

The simple *rubefacients* (such as camphorated
spirits and spirit of turpentine) are employed
chiefly with the view of exciting the action of the
cutaneous vessels, and may be applied daily over
a great part of the chest. They are of considerable use in an inactive state of the skin, accompanied with an irritable condition of the bronchial
membrane; they also often afford relief in slight
local pains. A sinapism, the strength of which
may be regulated according to the sensibility of
the skin, forms one of the most convenient and
effectual rubefacients.

Plasters, composed of burgundy pitch, and substances of a similar kind, may be ranked under
rubefacients, as they operate chiefly by exciting
irritation of the skin ; they also act by effectually
protecting the part from cold. When applied to
the back, they answer well, are less inconvenient

in that situation, and, moreover, leave the chest clear for other applications, such as sponging with salt water, vinegar and water, friction, &c.

Blisters. — After rubefacients, blisters are in most general use, and, when timely applied, they seldom fail to produce marked relief. In slight inflammations of the pleura, and in the catarrhal attacks of phthisical patients, blisters are of essential service, but when the case requires the abstraction of blood, either local or general, their application should, for the most part, be deferred until the practitioner is satisfied that the further employment of bleeding is unnecessary; this is the proper period for their use in the more acute cases. Even in catarrh, blisters should not be applied early in the disease, nor before the febrile excitement has been reduced; their effects are then very remarkable in removing the remains of the disease; whereas, if employed during the acute stage, they frequently increase the evil by the irritation which they excite: the prevailing error in the use of blisters is their too early application in the cases under notice.

A succession of blisters has been recommended in consumption, and when the skin is not irritable, and the patient does not suffer much incovenience from their operation, they are often useful; but when they excite much pain or irritation, they rarely do good; and in a disease which is attended with so many distressing symptoms, we ought not unnecessarily to aggravate them by the injudicious application of external irritants. When applied to persons who have a thin irritable skin, they should be covered with a piece of fine muslin, moistened with oil, and should be removed at the end of six or eight hours; in this way they will produce less irritation:—the less pain blisters give, and the fuller the discharge they occasion, the greater is the benefit derived from them.

Pustular Eruptions. — Tartar-Emetic Ointment has been of late more generally employed as an external irritant than any other application, and in general it answers well; although the sanguine expectations entertained of it by Dr. Jenner, who first employed this remedy, are, it is to be feared, far from having been realized.* Croton-oil has lately been used as an external irritant; it produces a slighter eruption than the tartar-emetic ointment, and is perhaps a more appropriate application over the trachea and larynx.

Issues and Setons.—A discharge of matter from the subcutaneous tissue, kept up for some time, has been long an esteemed remedy in consumption. Such artificial discharges may be considered general as well as local remedies, from their

* See his Letter to Dr. Parry on the Influence of Artificial Eruptions, &c.

influence on the general health, and may be useful in the state of tuberculous cachexia, before the deposition of tuberculous matter in the lungs ; and even after this has taken place, such discharges may have some effect in checking the progress of the disease. They are strongly recommended in this stage of the disease by Mudge. " In this critical and dangerous situation," says that judicious practitioner, "I think I can venture to say, from long experience, that, accompanied with change of air and occasional bleedings, the patient will find his greatest security in a drain from a large scapulary issue, assisted by a diet of asses' milk and vegetables."

The establishment of such discharges has in general been adopted in the advanced stage of consumption, when the measure could be of little utility and might do mischief. Issues are more particularly indicated in full gross habits of body, with little sensibility ; and if the patient has been subject to cutaneous diseases or ulcers, they will prove the more advantageous. In such cases they generally discharge freely, and give little pain ; and I agree with Mudge, that they should be large enough to ensure an abundant secretion. In irritable, sensitive, or spare persons with a thin skin, issues, or any other form of external discharge, will not prove of much use ; the irritation and distress which they occasion more than counterbalance any good effects

derived from them. Indeed, counter-irritants of all
kinds must be employed with considerable restrictions. When they excite little constitutional irritation, they are often beneficial; but, on the contrary, when they occasion much pain, increase the
action of the heart, or prevent sleep, we may be
well assured that their effects on the system will
be injurious.

In regard, therefore, to external applications and
discharges, I consider that, with due attention to the
restrictions laid down, considerable advantage may
be derived from their employment. They assist in
suspending the progress of the disease, while such
measures are adopted as are calculated to improve
the general health. Whoever expects more from
these remedies in consumption will, I believe,
be generally disappointed.

INHALATION. — The inhalation of volatilized
substances in the form of dry fumes and of watery
vapours has been supposed to be beneficial in consumption, from their being applied directly to the
seat of the disease.

Dry fumigations.—The inhalation of the fumes
of resinous and balsamic substances is a very ancient practice. From the time of Galen and Rhazes,
such fumigations have been employed in the treatment of pulmonary disease : they were particularly
advocated in this country by Bennet and Mead, but in
modern times they have gradually fallen into disuse.

It will not be necessary to go much into detail upon this practice, nor to dwell on the advantages which have been ascribed to it in the treatment of consumption. In chronic bronchial disease, or even in chronic tuberculous disease, the inhalation of gentle stimulants of this kind may be useful; but before we can decide on the particular cases to which they are applicable, we would require a series of experiments conducted by practitioners well acquainted with the nature of pulmonary diseases.

The only substance applied by fumigation which has attracted much attention in modern times is *Tar*. The vapour of tar was first recommended to notice by Sir Alexander Crichton, who was induced to try it by a conjecture of Mudge,—that the salutary effect of sea voyages is greatly assisted by the inhalation of an atmosphere impregnated with the volatile parts of the resinous and terebinthinate substances used in ships. The vapour is obtained by heating the tar over a spirit-lamp, a small proportion of subcarbonate of potass being previously added to neutralize any pyroligneous acid which the tar may contain. The heat should be moderate, and the vapour diffused in the chamber of the patient, which should be carefully maintained at an equable temperature. In some cases of pulmonary disease, accompanied with cough and expectoration, the beneficial effects of the tar-vapour appear to have been remarkable; while in others, which apparently were of a similar nature, it produced no sensible benefit, and was sometimes injurious by irritating the lungs or inducing hemoptysis. In the Appendix to the last edition of Sir Alexander Crichton's work, an account is given of some experiments made with this remedy in the hospital of La Charité at Berlin, by Drs. Hufeland and Neümann; wherein it is stated, " that of fifty-four patients, labouring under pulmonary consumption, four were cured, six, at their own request, left the hospital in a state of convalescence, sixteen did not receive any benefit from the remedy, twelve appeared to get worse under the treatment, and sixteen died."

I am not aware that in this country any well-conducted experiments on tar-vapour have been made on a large scale, except those of Dr. James Forbes, which were not in favour of it: one of its most injurious effects was to excite hemoptysis, which it did in many cases; and there is reason to believe that the general result of the trials has not been such as to encourage the continuance of the practice.*   Dr. Morton, of Philadelphia, gives the following favourable opinion of its efficacy. " After a fair trial with various substances, there is no one

---

* Remarks on Tar-Vapour as a Remedy in Diseases of the Lungs. Med. and Phys. Journ. Oct. 1822.

which I have prescribed in this form with equal success to tar in combination with subcarbonate of potash, in the manner recommended by Sir Alexander Crichton. In truth, I have seen it act like a charm." In chronic catarrh he knows of no plan of treatment that can vie with this. He also states that the tar fumigation was employed by the late Dr. Rush of Philadelphia, although in a different manner, upwards of thirty years ago.*

WATERY AND MEDICATED VAPOURS.—The inhalation of the steam of water, either pure or impregnated with emollient medicines, is also a practice of some antiquity. In cases of consumption attended with little expectoration, Bennet and others recommended the inhalation of the vapour arising from decoctions of emollient herbs; but this remedy was not much employed before the middle of the last century, when Mudge introduced it to notice as a cure for a catarrhous cough and inflammatory affections of the bronchial membrane.†
The apparatus which he employed for its inhalation, generally known by the name of " Mudge's inhaler,"

---

* For a full account of the effects of tar-vapour, and the mode of employing it, I beg to refer to Sir Alexander Crichton's sensible work, which, independently of the information it contains on this subject, will well repay the perusal.

† A Radical and Expeditious Cure for a Recent Catarrhous Cough, p. 131 et seqq.

is still in use, but it has been much improved by
Mr. Reid, the inventor of the stomach-pump.

The inhalation of warm vapour impregnated with
narcotic substances has been recommended as being
useful in allaying irritation of the mucous membrane
of the larynx and bronchi; but I am inclined to
believe that the chief benefit derived from the inhalation of medicated vapours has, in many cases,
been produced by the simple effects of the
vehicle. After trying various pectoral ingredi-
ents, Mudge found no vapour so inoffensive and
grateful to the lungs as the steam of simple warm
water. In a very irritable state of the bronchial
membrane, this author occasionally combined the
internal use of opiates with the warm inhalations,
and with good effect. When the air of a consumptive patient's room is very dry, the cough
frequently becomes more troublesome, and some
advantage is derived from a basin of warm water
placed near the patient; the vapour diffuses itself
in the air of the chamber, and renders it more
soothing to the irritated surfaces of the air-passages,
while it saves the patient the irksome la our of
inhaling.

CHLORINE.—About ten years ago M. Gannal, a
French manufacturer, having observed that consumptive patients experienced relief while breathing an atmosphere charged with the chlorine disen-

gaged in the manufacture of printed cottons, suggested it as a remedy for phthisis; and since that time numerous experiments have been made with chlorine in France and this country. M. Gannal, in several memoirs presented to the Academy of Medicine, relates numerous cases in which marked relief was obtained from its employment;* and a case is given by M. Cottereau, in which a cicatrix was found after death in a part of the lung where pectoriloquy and " gargouillement" were distinctly heard eighteen months before: the patient died of gastric fever.† Numerous other instances of the apparent success of the remedy have been recorded in the French periodical publications.‡ In this country, however, the trials made with chlorine have not been attended with the same beneficial results; it has frequently afforded great relief, but rarely effected a cure. I have tried it in many instances, and in several it has apparently suspended the progress of the disease; but the cases in which I employed it were in the advanced stage, when tuberculous cavities already existed in the lungs. Many of the cases recorded by others were also far advanced; and there can be little doubt that the cures related as having been effected by the inhala-

---

* See Potter's Translation of Gannal's Memoirs. Lond. 1830.

† Journ. Hebdom. t. ii. 1831.

‡ See Archives Générales de Médecine.

tion of chlorine occurred in persons whose lungs were diseased to a very limited extent only.

The inhalation of chlorine frequently relieves dyspnœa; in all the instances in which I found it beneficial, the freedom of breathing which it produced was one of its most obvious effects; in some cases it also appeared to allay the cough; in others I was compelled, by the irritation which it excited, to abandon its use; and in the majority of cases it produced no sensible amelioration.

The mode which I adopt in the use of chlorine is to direct the inhalation to be continued for five minutes only, and to be repeated frequently in the course of the day. A longer time fatigues the patient, and he returns to it with reluctance. I begin with five drops, and gradually increase the quantity to forty, but rarely go beyond this. The most convenient and efficient mode of inhaling chlorine would no doubt be to have it diffused in a room prepared for the purpose: the patient might enter occasionally, and respire the air impregnated with chlorine, as suggested by Mr. Murray.* The inconveniences which I have observed to arise from inhaling chlorine are soreness of the mouth and an increase of the bronchial irritation.

Of the inhalation of iodine I have no expe-

* A Treatise on Pulmonary Consumption, &c. by John Murray, F.S.A. F.L.S. &c. London, 1830.

rience.   M. Baudelocque found iodine exhibited
in this way totally useless in scrofula; while, administered internally and through the medium of
the skin, we have seen that it produced excellent
effects.   Hydrogen and carbonic acid gases, and
even oxygen and nitrous oxide, have been employed in consumption, but with no advantages to
entitle them to consideration.

When more correct views of the nature of consumption are generally entertained, we shall no
longer hear it asserted that the disease is to be
cured by inhalation or any other local means.
Such a practice is founded on erroneous views
of the nature of consumption, and is productive
of much mischief.   I do not, however, consider
local remedies as totally useless; on the contrary, I consider them valuable as palliatives,
and often of great service as adjuncts to those
measures which are directed to improve the condition of the general health and correct the tuberculous diathesis; but I decidedly condemn the
practice of relying on any local remedy as a principal means of curing a disease which originates
in and depends upon a morbid condition of the
whole system, and which can only be cured or
prevented by means directed to the improvement
of the general health.

SECT. III.—TREATMENT OF PARTICULAR SYMPTOMS.

COUGH.—Before employing any direct remedies to suppress the cough, it will be proper to examine into the cause of it, in order that we may adopt the most effectual means to palliate or remove it. If we find that it depends upon bronchial irritation, which is usually the case, the application of leeches over the lower part of the trachea, and rubefacients and blisters applied to the upper part of the chest, constitute the most efficient means of relief. If the cough originates in gastro-hepatic irritation and congestion, leeches to the epigastrium, and a few alterative doses of mercury with laxatives, will generally be found the best means of relieving it.

But at this early period of the disease the cough is seldom severe; it is not, in general, until the pulmonary disease has made considerable progress that this symptom becomes frequent and distressing. In addition to the general measures employed in the treatment of the disease, it will then be necessary to allay the cough, and procure sleep; with this view, narcotic medicines of the mildest kind should be tried before having recourse to opium, which, although one of the most valuable medicines in the treatment of consumption, should be used sparingly, and deferred, if possible, till a late period of the disease, in order that the patient may obtain the more benefit from it when its aid is most required. One of the common errors in the treatment of consumption is, in my opinion, a too early and too prodigal use of opiates in large doses : I often obtain the full effects of an opiate from four or five drops of the solution of the muriate of morphia without any subsequent inconvenience ;* indeed it is always desirable to begin with the smallest doses, because, as the disease advances, it is generally necessary to increase the quantity, for in the last stages it often becomes the chief solace of the patient amidst his multiplied sufferings. It is also advantageous, in many cases, to vary the preparation of opium. The pulvis ipecacuanhæ compositus is one of the best and most effectual medicines for allaying the cough.

When the cough is kept up by an accumulation of mucus in the bronchi, and there is much difficulty in expectorating, a gentle emetic will afford great and almost immediate relief, and may save the patient hours of harassing cough, and perhaps a restless night.

HEMOPTYSIS.—The pulmonary hemorrhage which attends the early stages of consumption, I believe to be in almost every case dependent upon con-

---

* The solution referred to is that recommended by Professor Christison of Edinburgh, (five grains of muriate of morphine to an ounce of distilled water;) it contains the same quantity of morphia as the tincture of opium of the Pharmacopœia.

gestion of the lungs, and hence I consider venesection the most effectual remedy. The quantity of
blood necessary to be abstracted must be regulated
by the urgency of the symptoms and the constitution of the patient; and when due attention is paid
to these circumstances, I believe that venesection
is always useful. Until the sanguineous congestion
of the lungs is diminished, and the increased
action of the heart, which generally attends active
hemorrhage, is somewhat abated, medicines given
with the view of suppressing the hemorrhage, will,
for the most part, produce little effect. I have
never had occasion to regret the employment of
bleeding, nor have I, in my own practice, observed
any evil consequences result from it. The quantity
of blood abstracted need not in any case be great;
but if the hemorrhage should return, and especially
if the excitement of the circulation should continue,
it may be necessary to repeat venesection several
times before the hemorrhagic action is subdued.
When there exists a disposition to frequent returns
of hemoptysis, small bleedings repeated from time to
time form the most effectual, and, in some cases, the
only means with which I am acquainted, of arresting the hemorrhage. A striking case illustrative
of the efficacy of this practice is recorded by Dr.
Cheyne in the fifth volume of the Dublin Hospital
Reports. As the gentleman was under my care in
Italy for some time before he became Dr. Cheyne's

patient, and as the case is altogether a very interesting one, I shall give some account of it.

This gentleman had been for many years subject to hemoptysis; but, after his return from the Continent in the autumn of 1824, it increased to such an extent that during four months he had from three to four attacks every day; and in the month of February, 1825, he was reduced to such a state of weakness and emaciation as to require assistance to be moved from his bed to a chair. It was in this condition, that, after having experienced the inefficacy of other remedies, Dr. Cheyne had recourse to frequent small bleedings. Six ounces of blood were taken from the arm, which had the effect of suspending the return of hemoptysis for four days, when a slight relapse occurred; the same quantity was again abstracted, and for ten days there was no return of hemoptysis. From this time three or four ounces of blood were regularly taken from the arm every week for a year, and once every month or six weeks for another year. During the first eighteen months of this practice, the blood was invariably cupped and buffy; after this time it presented the natural appearance. The pulse during the whole period of the complaint was never much accelerated; a most unpleasant sensation of weight was experienced in the chest in the recumbent posture. Another circumstance deserves notice:— the functions of the digestive organs, which had been ، constantly deranged during his illness, improved immediately after the bleedings were commenced and the hemoptysis was checked.

Having received a communication from this gentleman in October last, I am enabled to give an account of his health subsequently to Dr. Cheyne's report, (1827). With the exception of an occasional slight attack of hemoptysis, for which the lancet was used, he enjoyed good health till April, 1830, when the hemorrhage returned in a greater degree, and continued to recur frequently for two months, unchecked by bloodletting. When reduced to great weakness, he tried carriage exercise in the country, which appeared to be most beneficial in allaying the hemorrhage, and in the course of two months he was able to resume his clerical duties. In May, 1831, he had another attack, and again in December, 1832, since which time he has had no serious return, and has not used the lancet since December, 1833. At the date of his communication (October 8, 1834,) he was quite well, weighed between twelve and thirteen stone, was able to take much exercise on horse-back, and felt no inconvenience from reading the service and preaching twice on the same day.

There cannot be a stronger instance than this of the beneficial effects of small bleedings in suspending hemorrhage, and if this practice had not been so judiciously adopted by Dr. Cheyne, the patient

must inevitably have sunk under its continued recurrence. But in reviewing the history of the case,
I am disposed to think that the remedy was relied
on too exclusively, and the faith of the patient in
its efficacy was latterly somewhat shaken from its
failing to afford the usual relief during the last
attacks. I have little doubt that the abdominal
circulation was the primary seat of congestion in
this case: the early attacks of hemoptysis were
preceded by constipated bowels, pain in the region
of the liver, dyspepsia, headach, and depression of
spirits,—symptoms clearly indicative of congestion
of the vena portæ system.

The practice of small bleedings may, I believe,
be adopted with advantage in some other hemor-
rhages, as in hemorrhage from the bowels, me-
norrhagia, epistaxis, &c. I adopted the practice,
and with considerable benefit, in a case of obstinate hematemesis.

Local bleeding, especially by leeches, in the commencement of hemoptysis, or even when a congestive state of the lungs, with a disposition to hemoptysis, exists, is, in my opinion, a practice not free
from danger, and not unlikely to produce the evil
it is intended to remove or prevent. This was
exemplified in the case just recorded. While the
patient was at Rome, leeches were applied to the
anus, with the view of relieving abdominal plethora,
and before they had ceased to bleed, the patient

was attacked with pulmonary hemorrhage so violent as to require repeated venesection to subdue it. I have frequently observed the same effect, but in a slighter degree, to follow the application of leeches, and hence I consider the practice of abstracting blood in this manner from a plethoric person threatened with, or labouring under hemoptysis, apoplexy, or any other hemorrhage, not unattended with danger. In all cases where the object is to relieve congestion of the large vessels, general should, in my opinion, precede local bleeding. When, on the other hand, our object is to restore, or to promote a suppressed secretion, sanguineous or other, by the abstraction of blood, it is best done by leeches.

Various medicines have been used in the treatment of hemoptysis; some, from a belief in their specific powers in checking hemorrhage; others, from their power in diminishing the force of the circulation. When the action of the heart is increased, and more especially when there is reason to apprehend pulmonary inflammation, tartarized antimony combined with nitre forms one of the most efficient remedies; it is recommended by Dr. Cheyne as superior to all others " in cases of hemoptysis with inflammatory symptoms." A quarter, or even an eighth of a grain, with five to ten grains of nitre, every hour, is generally sufficient to abate the increased action of the heart and often to induce some nausea. Dr. Graves of Dublin places greater confidence in ipecacuan than any other remedy (after venesection). He gives two grains every quarter of an hour until there is some improvement, and then every half hour, or every hour, until the bleeding stops. Before he gives the ipecacuan, he prescribes a purgative injection and a saline purge—sulphate of magnesia, infusion of roses, and a little sulphuric acid.* The other remedies in most estimation in the treatment of hemoptysis are superacetate of lead, digitalis, nitre, sulphuric acid, and opium, the last of which is often useful after venesection, when there is much nervous irritation or alarm. I consider purgatives of great utility in pulmonary hemorrhage, which in the consumptive constitution is so frequently connected with hepatic congestion. I have, accordingly, often found that the returns of hemorrhage did not cease till the biliary secretion assumed a natural appearance; hence, in all cases of hemoptysis, I would recommend strict attention to the functions of the liver. Aperients of the least irritating kind deserve the preference; the saline laxatives generally

* Clinical Lectures, *Medical and Surgical Journal.*

To these lectures of Professor Graves I beg to refer for much valuable practical information. It is to be hoped that the Doctor will soon publish the result of his clinical observations in a different form.

answer best, and they need not prevent the exhibition of anti-hemorrhagic medicines.

I consider the application of cold water or ice to the chest a very doubtful measure; and the cold affusion over the whole body, which has been recommended, highly objectionable. Iced water or even small pieces of ice may be given internally with advantage. When hemoptysis has been checked by bleeding and other means, and there is danger of inflammation supervening, a blister will be beneficial in preventing this. Even during the continuance of the hemoptysis, blisters are often useful. When the loss of blood has been considerable, or if the patient's strength is much reduced, mild tonics may be employed with benefit as soon as the hemorrhage has ceased. In such cases, bark with sulphuric acid forms one of the best tonics. After an attack of hemoptysis, it is particularly necessary to watch the state of the pulmonary circulation; and when congestion of the lungs is indicated, a small bleeding, employed in season, may prevent a return of the hemorrhage. In chronic hemoptysis, unattended by any excitement of the circulation, and where a relaxed or debilitated state of the system exists, the preparations of iron prove the best remedies. Mead states that he found chalybeate mineral waters of great utility in chronic cases of consumption accompanied with hemoptysis, when taken daily for a long time in small quantities.* A more tonic diet may also be allowed in such cases.

I have entered rather fully into the subject of hemoptysis, because I consider it of great importance. The cure of pulmonary hemorrhage in persons threatened with consumption is not merely to be considered as the removal of a symptom; it may prevent the occurrence of consumption, if advantage is taken of the removal of pulmonary congestion to adopt such measures as shall obviate its return, and at the same time improve the general health. The presence of abdominal plethora in these cases must never be lost sight of; a strictly regulated diet, and attention to the functions of the chylopoietic viscera are absolutely necessary; as, unless we succeed in obviating abdominal plethora, pulmonary congestion and its consequences must ensue. The means by which this may be best effected have been already stated.

PAIN OF CHEST.—The pain which occurs during the progress of consumption is seldom very severe, unless it is complicated with acute pleuritic inflammation. The abstraction of a few ounces of blood by cupping, the application of leeches, or a blister, will generally be sufficient to remove it; but of all local applications I have found a sinapism the most

---

* Op. cit. lib. ii. cap. 2.

convenient and the most efficient in relieving the pains which accompany the latter stages of consumption. In persons of a very irritable state of skin, a warm poultice of linseed meal with a small proportion of mustard has considerable effect in mitigating pain without exciting much external irritation; friction with stimulating or opiate liniments, or the application of æther, will also often afford relief. When the pain is of a more fixed character, a slightly stimulating plaster may be applied with advantage. If these milder means fail, recourse must be had to a blister.

DYSPNŒA.—Difficult breathing, except during the last stage of the disease, does not generally cause much distress. During the paroxysms of oppressed breathing which occasionally occur at this period, a combination of æther and opium proves useful; and if they are very harassing, and the pulse admits of depletion, a small quantity of blood may be abstracted with advantage. Laennec recommends belladonna, but I have never seen it produce decided relief. In cases where the dyspnœa was constant, I have found the extract of stramonium, in small doses, a quarter or half a grain every day, very useful. External applications are sometimes beneficial, particularly when the difficult breathing returns in paroxysms; a mustard poultice is quickest in its operation, and may be applied either to the chest, arms, or feet. When the dyspnœa depends upon an accumulation of mucus in the bronchi, or a loaded stomach, an emetic will afford more relief than any other remedy : the inhalation of æther, or æther holding in solution some narcotic, is also occasionally useful; and in the last stage of the disease, when the oppression of breathing becomes very distressing, especially towards night, I have found opium and æther afford the most effectual relief.

NAUSEA AND VOMITING.—In a small proportion of phthisical cases, sickness of stomach forms a very distressing and obstinate symptom ; indeed, there is no symptom more difficult of relief.   I have known it prevail for years, the quantity of food retained during the whole time being incredibly small.   All the cases which I have seen, have occurred in young females of a strongly marked tuberculous constitution.   A strict adherence to a mild diet, the exclusion of every thing which is found by experience to irritate the stomach, and the use of food in the smallest quantity at a time, will often prevent or abate the vomiting.   In some cases I have seen decided benefit from the use of prussic acid, and in others from lime-water or liquor potassæ.   Seltzer water is also occasionally useful.   External remedies, such as sinapisms and blisters, produce temporary relief only.

HECTIC FEVER.—When hectic fever occurs in the early stages of consumption, and especially when it is accompanied with pain or tightness of the chest, it may be proper to have recourse to venesection; but in general small doses of tartarized antimony, combined with nitre, form the most appropriate remedy. During the hot stage, sponging the hands and feet with tepid vinegar and water will afford relief: but the cold fit frequently forms the principal and most distressing part of the febrile paroxysm. Bark occasionally relieves this stage, although its effects are for the most part only temporary. When the chill comes on at a particular time, its severity may often be abated by keeping the patient warmly covered in bed till the period of attack has passed. But the best means of controlling the hectic fever is a light and well regulated diet.

It was in the more chronic forms of hectic fever that Griffiths found his myrrh and steel mixture so useful. It is not easy to point out the circumstances under which it proves most beneficial. In chronic phthisis in old people I have often found this mixture, and chalybeates in other forms, produce excellent effects.

PERSPIRATION. — During the advanced stages of the disease the copious night perspirations of the consumptive patient form one of his most harassing symptoms. In many cases medicine has little power in diminishing these perspirations. Sulphuric acid is commonly used for this purpose; and when the debility is great, and there is no objection to its exhibition, advantage will often be derived from a combination of this acid with an infusion of bark, or with small doses of sulphate of quinine. When there are objections to the bark, infusion of sage may be advantageously made the vehicle for the acid; and the acetic may sometimes be substituted for the sulphuric acid. The most effectual plan of controlling the perspiration consists in regulating the patient's diet, which should be mild and moderate; and much warm fluid, particularly towards night, should be avoided. In the advanced stages of the disease the object is merely to diminish the perspiration; if we could stop it, it would not be proper to do so. When the perspirations are very copious, the patient should sleep in thin flannel or calico; and it is often necessary, and at all times a great comfort to him, to be rubbed dry with warm flannels, and to have the night-clothes changed.

DIARRHŒA.—Although the bowels are frequently irritable and easily deranged during the whole progress of consumption, diarrhœa does not in general occur in a severe degree till the advanced stage; before it appears, the expectoration is generally abundant, and the perspirations are copious. When diarrhœa occurs in the earlier stages, it often depends on an irritated and loaded state of the alimentary canal, produced by errors in diet or other accidental causes. In this case it will be remedied by gentle aperients, such as

rhubarb combined with carbonate of soda or magnesia ; and when the stomach is much oppressed,
an emetic may be premised with advantage : a
strict attention to regimen will generally prevent
its return under such circumstances. But when
the diarrhœa depends on ulceration of the mucous
follicles of the bowels, which, as I have already
shewn, is very generally the case, it becomes
severe and obstinate ; and we can easily understand how stimulants and rough astringents aggravate and increase it ; while a mild diet, consisting
chiefly of farinaceous food, such as rice, arrow-
root, and sago, with soups, milk, and a small proportion of the lightest animal food, diminish it,
add greatly to the patient's comfort, and may be
the means of prolonging his life. It is not sufficiently considered that the diarrhœa of the latter
stages of consumption depends upon diseased
bowels ; and that the almost constant existence of
intestinal ulcerations forbids the practice of loading
the stomach with large quantities of chalk mixture,
kino, catechu, and stimulating aromatics and exciting food, but rather calls for the employment of
a mild regimen and soothing medicines. Ipecacuan
in combination with some mild narcotic, or with
the compound ipecacuan powder, forms one of the
most useful remedies ; sulphate of copper is also
occasionally useful ; and an enema of starch and
opium frequently suspends the diarrhœa for a con-

siderable time, and produces sleep more effectually than any other remedy.

External applications, such as stimulating and opiate liniments, will often give relief to the uneasy sensation in the bowels which sometimes remains long after an evacuation. But the diarrhœa cannot be effectually relieved unless a strict adherence to the mildest diet is adopted; and the diet, likewise, ought to be of such a quality as to leave the smallest proportion of remora to pass through the bowels : at the head of such articles are arrow-root, sago, and rice. In chronic diarrhœa carriage exercise is often useful in abating the irritability of the bowels, and may often be employed with advantage for this purpose.

SECT. IV.—TREATMENT OF THE ADVANCED
STAGE.

As the disease advances, the case becomes in general more complicated, and consequently requires a corresponding variety of treatment. The extension of tuberculous disease in the lungs renders them less fitted for performing their functions, and they are more liable to congestion and inflammation; hence the increase of cough, dyspnœa, and pain,—symptoms which become more urgent as the disease of the lungs extends; the hectic fever, and especially the perspirations also generally increase; and the digestive organs, partly from sympathy, but more from the effects of tuberculous disease, become deranged, and nausea, vomiting, and still more frequently diarrhœa, add greatly to the patient's sufferings. According to the predominance of one or more of these symptoms must the means of relief be varied; hence the medical treatment of the advanced stages resolves itself chiefly into the relief of particular symptoms, a subject which has been considered in the preceding section. I would only observe that the patient's life may be prolonged, and the remaining term of his existence deprived of much of its discomfort and distress, by a strict adherence to a mild regimen, and by avoiding whatever excites the circulation or irritates the digestive organs. If these precautions are neglected, the hectic fever, perspirations, and diarrhœa increase; the patient's mind also becomes irritable under an exciting regimen, a circumstance which adds not a little to his own uneasiness, and is moreover most painful to the feelings of those around him: hence one great object of our treatment during the later stages should be to soothe and tranquillize both mind and body.

SECT. V.—TREATMENT OF VARIETIES AND
COMPLICATIONS OF CONSUMPTION.

Although the treatment of the different forms or
varieties of consumption is comprehended under
the general treatment already detailed, the peculiar
circumstances attending some of these forms require a brief notice.

ACUTE CONSUMPTION.—Of this, two varieties are
described. In the first, the violence of the disease
requires that the remedies should be applied with
corresponding activity. Bloodletting, emetics, and
whatever remedies the particular circumstances of
the case indicate, should be used in much quicker
succession than in ordinary cases of consumption.
In other respects the treatment does not differ from
that which is applicable to the disease in its more
ordinary form.

In the second variety of acute phthisis, the patient appears to sink rather from feebleness of constitution than the extent of disease; although in this
there is a deception, as the tuberculous disease of the
lungs often makes very considerable progress without
being indicated by the usual symptoms; and the pa
tient is far gone in consumption, when she is thought
to be merely threatened with it. In this case a regimen calculated to support the powers of the con-

stitution, and tonic medicines, are more strongly indicated, and are attended with more beneficial effects
than in the usual forms of the disease. Change of
air and a short voyage often produce good effects
in such passive forms of consumption, when the
patient has sufficient strength to bear the exertion
and fatigue necessarily attending such measures.

ACUTE FEBRILE CONSUMPTION.—On the treatment of this variety there is little to remark. The
nature of the symptoms and the rapid progress of
the disease scarcely leave a hope of benefit from
any mode of treatment. The disease bursts out at
once with violence, and its progress is generally
such as to bid defiance to all the resources of our
art: fortunately phthisis is rarely met with in this
form.

CHRONIC CONSUMPTION.—In this variety more
time is given for treatment, and if the disease is recognized in its early stage, the chances of checking
its progress and even of effecting a cure are much
greater than in the more acute forms of the disease.
Local remedies, such as blisters and issues, may
be employed with greater freedom and advantage,
and a long sea-voyage and change of climate are
often admissible and highly useful in chronic consumption, even when the lungs are tuberculous to
an extent which would forbid such a measure in
the usual form of the disease.

BRONCHIAL CONSUMPTION.—The treatment of this form of consumption differs little from that of the disease in its usual form: indeed the difficulty of ascertaining whether the tuberculous disease is confined to the bronchial glands is a reason why it can be rarely treated as a distinct form of the disease. When there is reason to believe that it is so confined, or that the disease is chiefly limited to these glands, the good effects of iodine in the diseases of the external lymphatic glands warrant a cautious trial of it.

The neck, the upper parts of the chest and back should be particularly well protected with flannel at all times; but irritating applications to these parts should be avoided: if counter-irritation or a local discharge is considered advisable to the case, the arm will be the best place for either application. A well-regulated diet, great attention to maintain a regular state of the bowels and a free biliary secretion, warm clothing, and a residence in a mild, dry air, constitute the essential part of the treatment. Children labouring under tuberculous cachexia, or incipient tuberculous disease, whatever may be its site, derive great benefit from a change to a warm climate;— a residence of two or three winters in the south of Europe will do more to promote the effects of a proper regimen in correcting the tuberculous constitution than any other means with which I am acquainted.

COMPLICATIONS.—The treatment of the various diseases which complicate consumption in its progress, such as laryngeal irritation and ulceration, inflammation of the bronchi and lungs, &c. does not differ from that usually employed in the same diseases when idiopathic. It must, however, be borne in mind that they are merely complications, and must be treated with caution proportioned to the advanced state of the tuberculous disease and the debility of the patient.

There is one of these affections,—chronic inflammation and ulceration of the larynx, which deserves particular attention, as, although very often merely a complication of tuberculous disease of the lungs, it is occasionally idiopathic, and requires to be treated accordingly.*

SECT. VI.—REGIMEN.

The great difficulty of directing the regimen of persons of a tuberculous constitution consists in the discrepancy between the wants of the system and the powers of the assimilating organs. The former

---

* For an account of this disease and the various other diseases which may be mistaken for or confounded with consumption, with their treatment, I beg to refer the reader to Dr. Abercromby's valuable papers on the *Pathology of Consumptive Diseases*, in the Edinburgh Med. and Surg. Journal, vol. xvii and xviii.

appears to call for a strongly tonic diet; while its employment rarely fails to aggravate the weak and irritable condition of the latter, and to depress still further the powers of the constitution: hence it is evident that the food best adapted to the digestive organs, is that which will ultimately contribute most effectually to the strength of the system. The disregard of this obvious law of the economy has given rise to the diversity of opinion which still prevails respecting the regimen of consumptive and scrofulous patients. I have already stated my opinion on the diet of children, and have alluded to the prevailing error of over-feeding young persons of a strumous constitution.

During the early stage of consumption the diet ought to be mild, and where there is a tendency to pulmonary congestion or inflammation, it should be strictly antiphlogistic; but the diversity of the prevailing symptoms renders it impossible to lay down any general rule. I would simply remark that when, from any cause, it is necessary to reduce the diet, its subsequent increase should be made with great caution and very gradually.

As consumption advances, the diet must be regulated according to the circumstances of each case: one person will bear, and derive advantage from, a diet which in another would excite fever: any general rule, therefore, would be weakened by so many exceptions as to make it almost useless. Too much

importance is generally attached to the food, and too
little consideration given to the state of the digestive
organs; and hence it is erroneously supposed that
the emaciation and wasting of the patient may be
checked by an additional quantity and richer quality of food; by which the stomach and bowels
are disordered, and a new train of symptoms induced,
which complicate the case, and add to the patient's
distress.

Although a mild diet is most generally suited to
the advanced stages of consumption, cases occur in
which it is advisable to adopt a more exciting regimen; and instances are on record where consumptive patients, after long lingering under a spare diet,
have rapidly improved in strength, and have been
apparently cured by a diet of an opposite quality.

The patients who have been cured in this manner
were no doubt persons in whom the tuberculous
disease of the lungs was very limited, and advancing
to a cure before the change of regimen was adopted;
and were probably indebted as much to the preceding course of mild diet as to the subsequent use of
an exciting regimen. In consumption, even when
of a chronic character, a change from a mild to a
stimulating diet would often do mischief, and interfere with the curative process going on in the lungs,
and this is much more frequently the case than the
reverse; indeed the proportion of cases is very
small in which a stimulating regimen will prove

useful. When adopted, much judgment and discernment on the part of the practitioner will be necessary in deciding on the proper period for its employment, the extent to which it should be carried, and the modifications which it requires in individual cases. When such a change of diet is made, it should generally be accompanied by an increase of exercise in the open air.

The cases likely to be cured by the stimulating plan of treatment,—by the beef-steak-and-porter system,—bear so small a proportion to those which would be injured by it, that I do not consider it deserving of further notice. Many more patients have been preserved by the early adoption of a milk and vegetable diet, with a residence in the country; and the instances are numerous in which this regimen, adopted in the commencement of tuberculous disease, proves more serviceable than any other. The jelly of some of the mosses forms a nutritious article of diet well suited to some consumptive patients: the Iceland moss jelly has been generally preferred; it affords a light form of nourishment, and its bitter qualities render it useful in a languid state of the stomach. Asses' milk and goats' whey are well-known articles of diet in such cases, but it is unnecessary to go into detail on this part of the subject, as every medical practitioner is acquainted with it.

When a cure or a suspension of consumption has been effected, the utmost attention will be necessary on the part of the patient to prevent a renewal of disease in the lungs. While his mode of living is the most favourable for the maintenance of his general health, it is also essential to his well-being that he should avoid, with the most sedulous care, whatever is likely to produce congestion or irritation of the respiratory organs. The power of fully expanding the chest is diminished, and the capacity of the lungs reduced, by adhesions of the pleura and by the destruction of a portion of the lungs. The pulmonary circulation is therefore less free, and unless the quantity of nourishment and degree of bodily exercise are adapted to such diminished capacity of the respiratory organs, inflammation or hemorrhage will most likely be the consequence. Every indication of internal irritation or congestion in such a person should receive immediate attention, more especially when the chest is the part affected. The state of the digestive organs also requires particular attention; abdominal congestion soon leads to a similar condition of the lungs, and under such circumstances the patient's life is placed in imminent danger: he may be carried off by pulmonary hemorrhage or inflammation in the course of a few days. By avoiding, as much as possible, all causes of mental excitement, by a strict adherence to a mild and rather abstemious diet, by attention to the functions of the digestive organs and of the skin, by gentle but much exercise in the open air, and, above all, exercise on horseback, the lives of such persons may be long preserved in a state of comfort.

A residence in a mild climate for some years will greatly promote the restoration of the general health, and tend to prevent a recurrence of disease in the lungs.

THE END.